THE LUNG

MONKEY PRESS takes its name from the Monkey King in 'Journey to the West', the sixteenth century classical novel by Wu Chengen. The story narrates the bringing of Buddhist scriptures to China; a journey which involves many misadventures and opportunities for learning. The incisive obervations of Monkey are humourously contrasted with the sometimes misplaced compassion of Tripitaka, the monk under his protection. Monkey blends vision, wisdom and insight with irreverence and mischief.

CHINESE MEDICINE FROM THE CLASSICS

Essence Spirit Blood and Qi

The Seven Emotions

The Eight Extraordinary Meridians

The Way of Heaven: Neijing Suwen chapters 1 and 2

The Secret Treatise of the Spiritual Orchid

The Kidneys

The Lung

The Liver

Spleen and Stomach

The Heart in Ling shu chapter 8

Heart Master Triple Heater

THE LUNG

Claude Larre and Elisabeth Rochat de la Vallée

transcribed and edited by Caroline Root

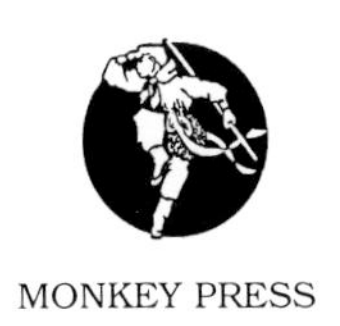

MONKEY PRESS

CHINESE MEDICINE FROM THE CLASSICS: THE LUNG

Claude Larre and Elisabeth Rochat de la Vallée

ISBN 1 872468 01 2

Transcribed from a seminar organised by Peter Firebrace, February 1987

Text Editor: Caroline Root

Production and Design: Sandra Hill

Calligraphy: Qu Lei Lei

Printed on recycled paper by Spider Web, London N7

CONTENTS

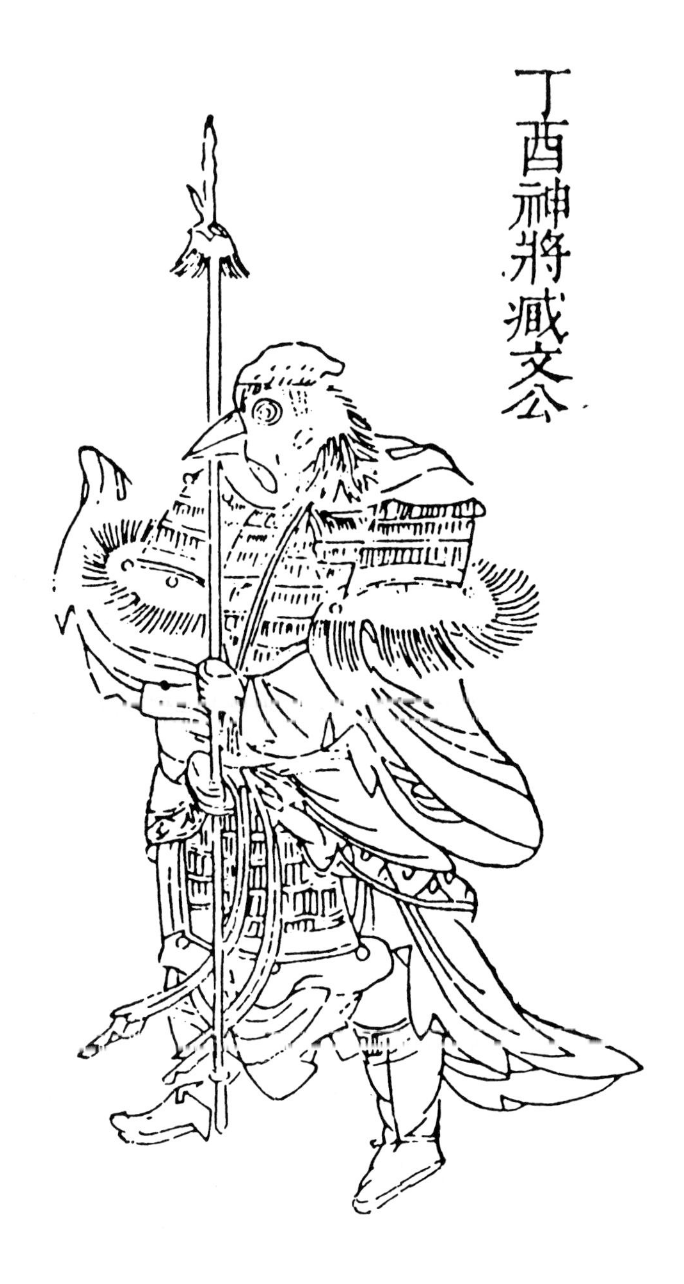

'One does the cock' p.10

FOREWORD

The evolution of Chinese medicine in the West has been hampered by the lack of access to the original texts of the Huangdi Neijing and the illuminating commentaries that have expanded on its seminal ideas down the centuries. Without this access many students are restricted to the modern version, 'Traditional' Chinese Medicine (TCM), sometimes without the appreciation that this is definitely an edited version, since it has been subjected not only to the censorship of a political regime, but also cleaned up and dressed down for scientific respectability. The irony is that real modern science is moving back to qualities, fields, interrelations, energy and the void - away from the dead-end of strict logic and overrationality to the dynamics and interplay of heaven/earth/man. TCM has much to offer and has established a basic level of theory and practice, but it is not the whole story by any means. As Ted Kaptchuk writes in his introduction to 'The Fundamentals of Chinese Medicine' by the East Asian Medical Studies Society (Paradigm Press 1985):

'Idealist' 'feudal', 'incomplete', 'unclear', 'inaccurate' 'metaphysical' and 'primitive' ideas that did not fit into the acceptable dialogue were omitted. Traditional Chinese Medicine was to be a neat and rational set of theories and practices.

The present series of seminar transcripts is therefore offered as a refreshing dip, but not only into the distant past, with its world of seedling images, the coded, concentrated power of the ideograms and their skilful interweaving in the early texts, where sequence and structure themselves embody meaning. For this is not just an historical study, not some dry, academic, overintellectual appraisal of an antiquated medical system. It is vitally relevant to the present and future, not just of Chinese medicine, but of medicine as a whole. The rapidly growing systems of herbalism and homeopathy - as well as acupuncture - are, for example, all based on an understanding of 'mutual resonance', a key concept in Chinese philosophical and medical texts. Paul Unochuld in the introduction to his translation of the Nan Jing, Classic of Difficult Issues (University of California Press 1986) has called Chinese medicine *the medicine of systematic correspondance.* 'Resonance' gives less implication of a fabricated system and more that of a discovery of a naturally occuring phenomenon. It is not an imposed order which has been artificially created - specific harmonics naturally resonate from a fundamental. Each homeopathic remedy resonates with a specific symptom picture. As the texts unfold, the *qi* resonates - through direction, climate, element, taste, organ, body part, etc - an expression of the same quality or essence manifesting at successive levels.

The aim of this series is to deepen and enrich our understanding of Chinese medicine. It is intended to be used alongside more readily available material, not to replace it. The classics are full of potent teaching, itself a catalyst for change. In this series of seminars we have been fortunate to share the knowledge of Claude Larre and Elisabeth Rochat de la Vallée, of the Ricci Institute, European School of Acupuncture (Paris). Their work on the medical classics now spans almost two decades and that work itself is founded on a deep understanding of the philosophical texts behind them - Lao zi, Zhuang zi, Lie zi, Huainan zi and others. They combine methodical scholarship with a sensitive ability to weave the diverse threads of this deep and subtle subject into a coherent whole, so revealing its inherent simplicity. Their work speaks for itself and will provide a strong and reliable basis for those interested in the theory and practice of Chinese medicine.

Peter Firebrace
London 1989

FOREWORD TO THE SECOND EDITION

It is over ten years since the first edition of this book was published. The social, political and academic contexts in which Chinese medicine is studied and practised have changed considerably. During this time a well-trained and organized profession has emerged and there is a high level of public acceptance. A very wide range of original source material is now available in English translation, along with innumerable commentaries on and interpretations of the theory and practice of Chinese medicine.

The great pleasure and value to be found in the work reprinted here (in a re-edited version with the relevant Chinese characters inserted into the text) is that it roots our understanding and experience of Chinese medicine in simple yet profound and perceptive explanations of the movement of life. The gift to us of the work done over thirty years by Father Larre and Elisabeth Rochat de la Vallée is that it is authentic in the highest sense of the word: authoritative, faithful, genuine and true. It is rooted in the classics, retained and held firmly in the classics, and possessed of a clear vision of the place of humanity within the universe. Thus grounded the authors are able to range freely in their explanations and observations never losing sight of the essential truth that all life is movement, originates in movement and without movement is dead.

Caroline Root 2001

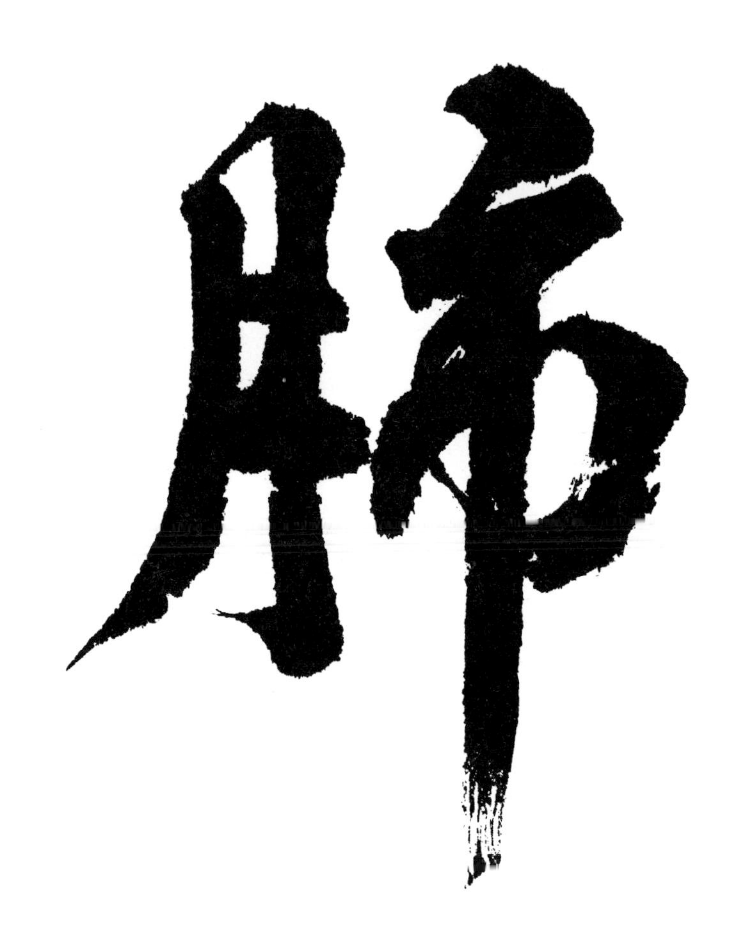

fei, the lung

THE IDEOGRAM FOR THE LUNG

Elisabeth Rochat: When we studied the spleen and stomach we were able to grasp an idea of their functions from the ideograms of their names. With the lung and metal it is not exactly the same situation. It is more complicated to show the movement and characteristics of metal from the Chinese texts, or to grasp the function of the lung from the ideogram. So we will try to use other ways to understand the lung, autumn and metal, and the very specific function of the lung inside the body.

The ideogram for the lung, *fei* (肺), is made with the radical for flesh. You can find the etymology in Weiger lesson 79G. The other part of the ideogram is a representation of plants branching up from the soil, part of the ideogram for earth, *tu* (土), is contained in it, but without the lower horizontal line. It is not an image of plants which stand up straight from the soil but of creeping plants which spread out, multiplying indefinitely. By extension this ideogram also has the meaning of multiplication or something like fibres, and I think it is like an anatomical aspect of the lung, which is why it was chosen for the ideogram of the lung. It is impossible to interpret this ideogram any more than that, but we can show some others with the same construction with another radical.

If we add the radical for general vegetation to the upper part we then have an ideogram with the meaning of bushy vegetation providing shade. If we add the radical for rain we have the idea of rain falling with great heaviness. The idea of something luxuriant, for example, luxuriant vegetation, can always be found in this right-hand part of the character. It appears in the ideogram for south, with some transformation, because the south is the area of very luxurious vegetation. Sometimes you can find the same ideogram with the pronunciation *shi* meaning a market, a place for exchange, and according to Su wen chapter 52, this market, *shi*, is a special name for the stomach. This is quite unconnected with the ideogram's other meaning of bushy, creeping vegetation.

SU WEN CHAPTER 2

The three months of autumn are called
overflowing and balancing.
The *qi* of heaven becomes urgent.
The *qi* of earth is resplendent

One retires early, one rises early.
One 'does the cock'.
Exerting the will peacefully and calmly,
to soften the repressive effect of autumn.
Gathering in the spirits and storing up the *qi*.
Pacifying the *qi* of autumn,
without letting the vitality be scattered outside.
Making the *qi* of the lung clear and fresh.
This is the way that is proper to the *qi* of autumn,
which thus corresponds to the
maintaining and gathering-in of life.

To go counter-current would injure the lung,
causing diarrhoea in winter through
an insufficient contribution to storage.

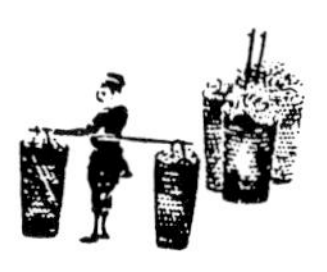

SU WEN CHAPTER 2: AUTUMN

Elisabeth Rochat: We can begin with two chapters of the Su wen, chapter 2 and chapter 5. In chapter 2 there is a description of the characteristics of autumn, and what the movement of life and vitality is like during this period of the year. In chapter 5 there are all the connections with the west, metal, the lung and so on, and with all the parts of the body which represent this movement.

Claude Larre: The ideogram for autumn, *qiu* (秋), is made up of two parts. On the left the character is the same as *mu* (木), wood, but with an extra stroke on the top giving the meaning of a stalk with an ear. Usually the ear of grain comes at the end of summer but if you push that a little further you come to autumn. On the right side the character is *huo* (火), fire, so the combination of these two makes *qiu* (秋), autumn. This is the opposite of *chun* (春), spring. We understand that at the end of winter the power of the sun is lower, is under the ground, so the plant pushes up. In autumn, on the other hand, there is no more pushing upward, there is only the bringing to maturity of the same plant which you saw in spring. The correspondence between spring and autumn is so strong that you can say *chun qiu* to mean a period of time and the Chunqiu zuozhuan is the fifth book in the collection of the Five Classics. It is a chronicle which describes the relationships of the state of Lu, the state of Confucius, with all the other states around it. But *chun qiu* has a larger meaning than just chronicle, it is for any period of time.

Elisabeth Rochat: In the seasons we can see the unfolding and progress of time, and time is nothing other than a succession and movement of different qualities of *qi*, the specific movement of *qi*. And the same succession and movement of *qi* occurs inside the human body in order to organize and maintain life. Spring is between winter and summer, this is obvious, but the meaning for the Chinese is that the root of spring is in winter, and its direction and expansion is towards summer. In spring you can begin to go out, but not too strongly and not without some precautions and so on. If you look at the liver in the human body, the root is *yin* (陰), in the essences and blood and in the kidneys, and the movement, direction and expansion of this effect are *yang* (陽), in the springing up and out of *qi*.

With autumn we have exactly the opposite; it is between summer and winter, with its root in summer and its tendency and direction towards winter. In the lung we see the same double aspect as with the liver, with the movement of expansion and circulation right up to the extremities of skin and body hair, but also the concentration and descending movement. We can see these two seasons, spring and autumn, as a hinge or pivot.

The three months of autumn are called overflowing and balancing

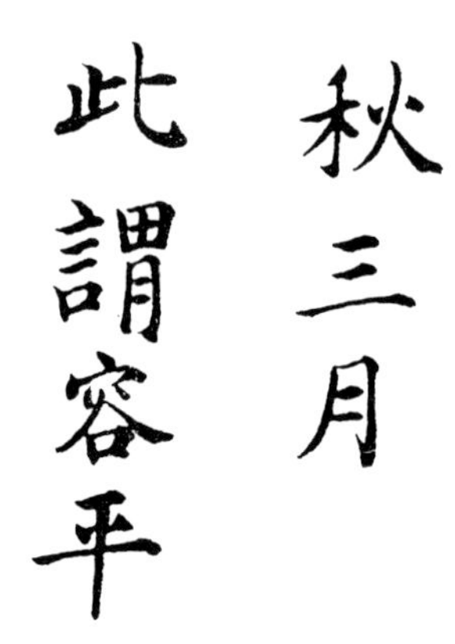

In overflowing we have the effects of summer, when all the cereals and fruits are completely achieved and it is time for harvest. With balancing, *ping* (平), you can see the meaning from the character. This is very important because we find the idea of equilibrium (though not exactly this ideogram) in the functioning of the lung. *Ping* means to restore the good balance between all sorts of *qi*. It is also to be very strong and to cut off anything which goes beyond the limit. Autumn is the time for punishment when you cut the cereal crops or cut off the heads of criminals. In the Book of Rites, another of the Five Classics, it says that autumn puts everything back in the balancing scales.

Claude Larre: Everything has to be measured exactly in order that all the trades and exchanges in the country are according to the true value. The capacity, the volume and the value of gold and silver or whatever has to be verified. It means that autumn has to be strict and exact, and the balance is between *yin* and *yang*.

Elisabeth Rochat: In the summer you can cheat a little bit, but not in autumn! We will see the same thing with the lungs which receive all the *mai* (脈), the network of animation of the body, at the morning audience and restore equilibrium at dawn. At this time you can see the pulse in very good balance.

Claude Larre: Elisabeth is referring to the fact that every morning all the officials go to the court in order to be assigned different tasks, and every morning the one hundred *mai* or *mo* have to go to the court in order to be regularized and to take their charges anew so that everything starts right each morning. This image of going to the court in the morning is an expression from the text and not from our own imagination.

The qi of heaven becomes urgent

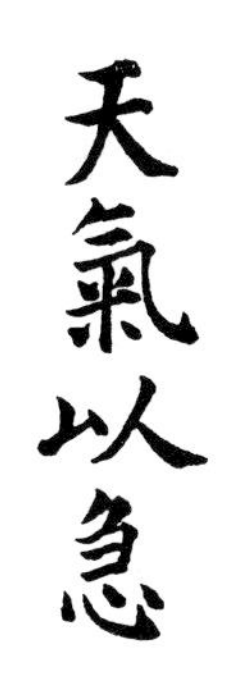

Elisabeth Rochat: The *qi* of heaven which is clear, has the effect of pressing downwards, exerting a pressure, as though it is withdrawing into the interior. This interior can be the interior of the living being or the interior of heaven. Therefore, for this reason during winter the *qi* of heaven retires into the bosom of itself and has nothing to do with earth, so the winter is the time of separation. On the other hand this *yang*, clear *qi* of heaven has to go into the depths of the body, following this same movement. There is no difference between the movement that penetrates to the depths of your being and that which rises up into the depths of heaven.

Claude Larre: Your own self is made from the purest energy from heaven, so while heaven does that, you are doing the same with heaven.

Elisabeth Rochat: Autumn is the period during which the normal movement of spring and summer is reversed. During spring and summer the *yang qi* goes towards the exterior in an expansion from the interior, and the *yin* is like the basis or foundation of that. During the autumn we have to reverse this, and the exterior is the property of the *yin qi*, while the *yang qi* of life is secure in the depths of the body.

For this reason autumn is the great period for intermittent fevers with the alternation of cold and warmth, because there can be some blockage and this movement does not happen correctly. But you can also have the same cold and warmth in spring. Then the name in the ancient texts is not exactly the same, they are called tepid diseases. Here the blockage is in the other movement with the *yang* spreading to the exterior.

The qi of earth is resplendent

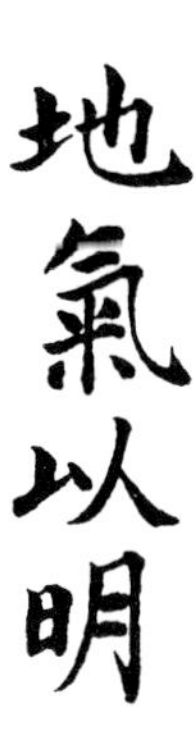

In autumn earth is very rich and bears all the fruits, it is very powerful and shows all the shapes and forms that earth can give.

One retires early,
one rises early

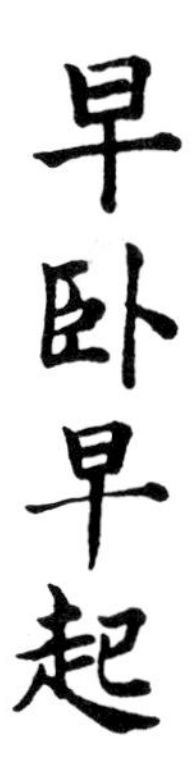

This is following the sun and warmth, but in autumn we have to rise less early because the warmth and the sun are receding. One retires early because during the evening and night the coolness arrives early.

One 'does the cock'

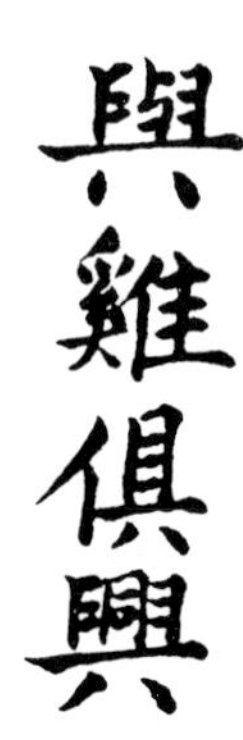

This is an expression used to describe the situation in which a living or human being is *yin* outside and *yang* inside. This is because, especially in Daoist books, a very strong fighting cock, is not a cock of great aggression on the outside but is very calm and still. But if this cock has to fight another cock he is the fastest and he wins because all his force comes out from the inside without a blockage.

Claude Larre: All martial arts are like that, you have your strength inside and you are quiet, just making your decision to move when it will have most effect.

Exerting the will peacefully and calmly, to soften the repressive effect of autumn

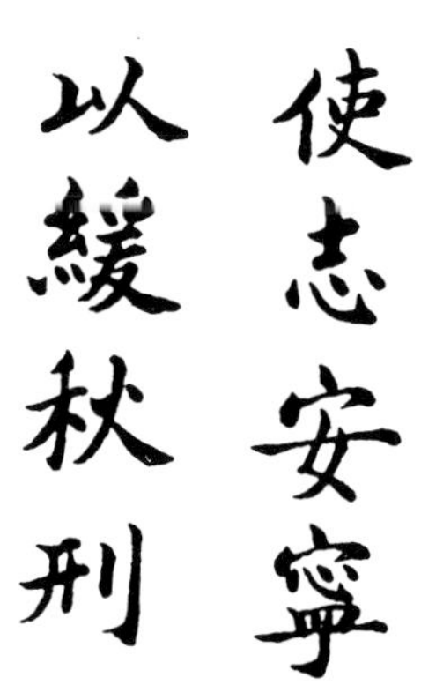

Elisabeth Rochat: The repressive effect of autumn is double in nature. It is not only the period of harvest or the period of maturation of all things, it is also, in the second period of autumn the time in which all vegetation begins to wither and shrivel. Harvest is the beginning of this time when the earth becomes bare, and in human society autumn is the time for punishment when criminals go to jail or to the place of execution. But it is necessary not to have any violence and to be very calm and peaceful at the same time as you are cutting off people's heads!

The violence of life is more present in the spring because it is a movement where *yang* can be visible, while in autumn *yang* can slowly become more invisible inside the depths of the body. For this reason acting peacefully and calmly you can soften the repressive effect of autumn, because in acting violently you will produce a countercurrent to the natural flow of life.

Gathering in the spirits
and storing up the qi

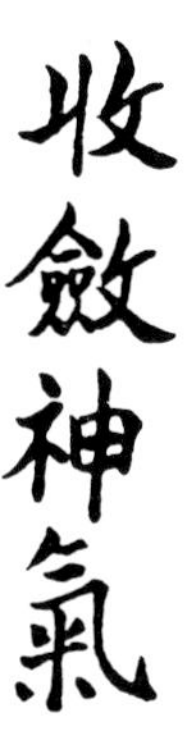

Elisabeth Rochat: This is the time of harvest, but not only for the cereals and grains which must be put in the granaries for the winter to avoid starvation. If you want to survive winter it is also necessary to store spirits and *qi* in your own internal granaries. *Qi* is the *yang* of life, the dynamism, vitality and movement of life, and spirits preserve the good direction of life within you. You have to protect the vitality in yourself, and the most important aspects of it are the spirits and the *qi*.

Pacifying the qi of autumn,
without letting the vitality
be scattered outside

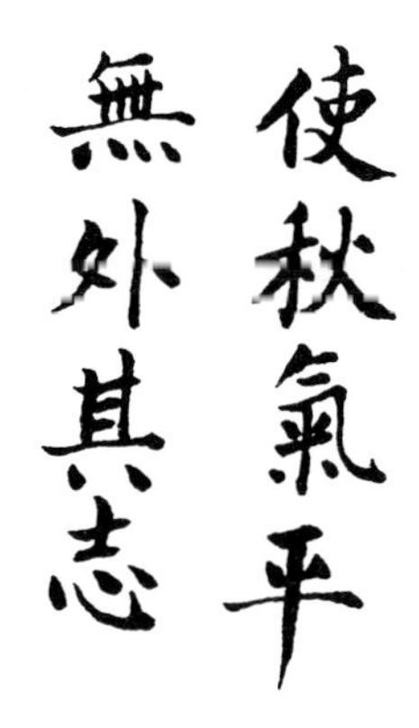

This is the same idea, that autumn is the period of cleaning out. During the spring and summer you can have strange ideas, and you can say something against the government quite easily, but not in autumn! In autumn you have to concentrate all the force of your ideas and being for the rigours of winter, because winter is the period of danger. You streamline yourself, and you have to follow the party line because it is the only way to survive. We have to keep the vitality inside, which is the contrary of summer when we can sweat. It is not very good to sweat in autumn and especially not as autumn nears winter, because this is a way in which vitality in one form can go outside the body, and you risk creating a deficiency. This is to be avoided. The word pacifying means to put in good equilibrium and balance. You know that in the past France and England have pacified various countries around the world, which means we were just bringing a good balance to them! Sometimes it can be with the same effect as autumn!

Making the qi of the lung clear and fresh

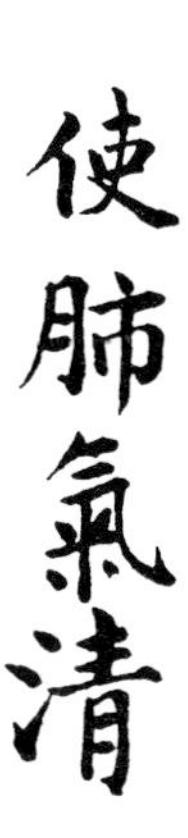

The ideogram for clear and fresh is *qing* (清). The *qi* of the lung has to be *qing*. It has to be clear because it is the *qi* of heaven and the subtle essence of alimentation, and it has to be fresh because if dryness or warmth are in excess then the lung is in a very difficult position. You know that unclear, troubled energy can bring a lot of disease. So during autumn it is especially important that the lung, which is like the *qi* of heaven in the human body, is really clear, and that the clear *qi* is rising and expanding. A second idea is that heaven's *qi* is the clearest that you can imagine, and its movement and activity is just to descend to earth. If this did not happen there would be no way to make heaven and earth have communication. The lung and the *qi* of the lung have to be the clearest inside the body with the double function of expanding and diffusing, and the only way for the upper part to act is to descend.

This is the way that is proper to the qi of autumn
which thus corresponds to the maintaining and gathering
in of life. To go counter-current would injure the lung

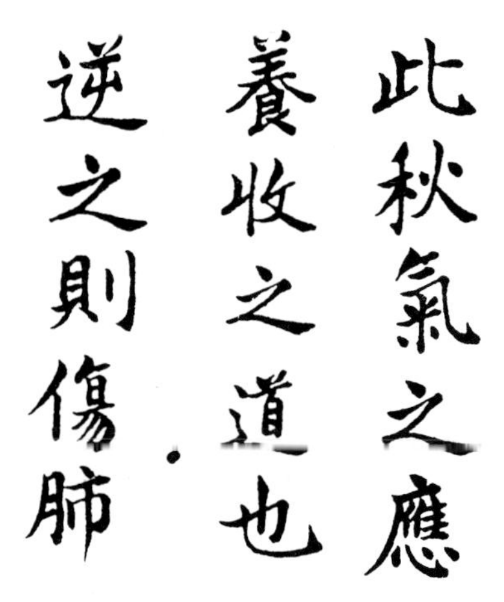

The lung is exactly the same expression of movement, with the same quality of *qi* inside the body, as autumn is in the progression of seasons.

Causing diarrhoea in winter through an insufficient contribution to storage

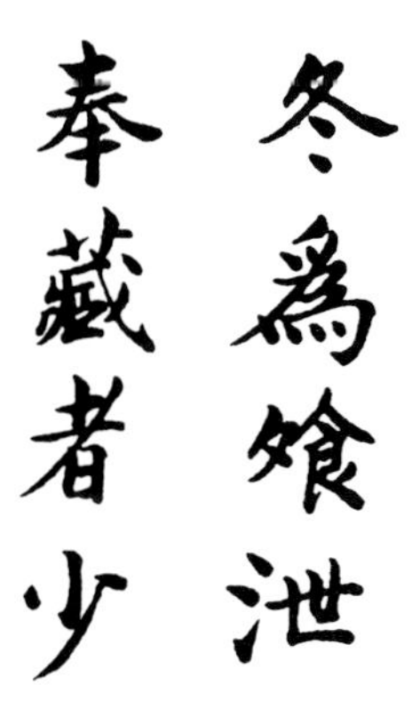

If during autumn or if through the lung you are unable to gather in and harvest, in winter it will be worse. There will not only be a lack of the gathering in but there will also be a loss in the form of diarrhoea because you are unable to retain the vitality and essences. Everything passes through the body without profit because in this situation you can imagine the middle heater (spleen and stomach) is weak and cannot ensure good digestion. So this kind of diarrhoea is with undigested food, and as a result you are unable to grasp the essences and nourishment necessary for the maintenance and rebuilding of life.

Claude Larre: This is a special point for chronological biology. The thing has to be seen from two aspects. One is now, what happens if you are not doing what is proper to the season? The other is that in Chinese teaching if in autumn, you are not doing what you should be according to the laws of the season, then you must expect that in the next season, winter, the organs which are supposed to work then will not have been made ready so there is a lack of preparation and support. When Elisabeth was talking about the lungs she said that if in autumn you were not abiding by the laws of autumn, then you would have bad effects in autumn, and when winter comes you would be in a state of weakness and would have diarrhoea.

Elisabeth Rochat: What are the characteristics of autumn? Autumn must have munificence and overflowing, but at the same time carefully avoid all excitation or agitation. So the season which is able to show this overflowing is also able to keep without letting the vitality be scattered outside. It can put boundaries and limits on itself and can begin the movement of returning to storing.

Autumn is the season that can produce this overflowing and abundant vegetation and cereals with all their splendid munificence as well as being able to put limits on its vitality so that it does not scatter outside. It is a balancing, and we see that especially with the lung which is able to send *qi* out to the skin and to stop any overflowing, so there is no loss. We will see later that this is a good aspect of the rhythm with which lung and metal and autumn are connected.

SU WEN CHAPTER 5

The western quarter gives rise to dryness,
dryness gives rise to metal,
metal gives rise to the acrid taste,
the acrid taste gives rise to the lung,
the lung gives rise to the skin and body hair,
the skin and body hair give rise to the kidneys,
the lung masters the nose.

In heaven it is dryness, on earth it is metal
Among parts of the body it is the skin and body hair,
among the *zang* it is the lung,
among colours it is white,
among notes it is *shang,*
among sounds it is sobbing,
among movements which react to change it is to cough,
among the orifices it is the nose,
among the tastes it is acrid,
among expressions of willpower it is grief.

Grief injures the lung,
joyful excitement prevails over grief.

SU WEN CHAPTER 5: THE FIVE ELEMENT RESONANCES

Elisabeth Rochat: The ideogram for west is *xi* (西). It is the beautiful image of a bird resting on its nest. (Weiger Lesson 41D)

Claude Larre: With the character for east, *dong* (東), it is not a question of a bird but of the sun. Yet the sun transforms itself into a bird at the end of its course to the west according to the Chinese. So for them there is no difference between the sun and the bird, they both are in the air and the bird exemplifies the *yang* power of earth and the sun exemplifies the *yang* power of heaven. It starts its life as the sun and finishes its life as a bird sitting on its nest, and this is seen in the characters. Ultimately, if we are not relating to vegetation or what we see in the sky, but are relating to what is behind all that, they are the same thing. That is typical of the Chinese scheme of things.

Elisabeth Rochat: The west is the region of the sunset, and at sunset birds go to roost. We can see from this ideogram and from the etymology that in the idea of west there is a movement of return. In the quality of the *qi* of the west you will find the same quality of *qi* as in autumn, there is something urgent, a concentration and a gathering. We saw that autumn has the munificence of harvest as well as the threat of bareness, and it is the same thing in the west with the sunset. At the moment of sunset there is an overflowing of light, but at the same time it is the beginning of night, of darkness and cold.

Each region and direction of space has a particular deity or genie, and the genie of the west is also the genie of punishment. He has the face of a man and the claws of a tiger, with white body hair. Another important thing is that in Chinese legends the west is the special region for spirits. The traditional explanation is that the spirits search for a dwelling place where peace, balance and equilibrium are good and where all cleaning up has been done. In such a place the spirits can have a rest full of serenity.

Claude Larre: The fact is that the Chinese are more concerned with peace than ourselves, and they know that the spirits would be miserable if they went to a place where things are not tidy and where there was nothing to eat. So since the west is a well-balanced region it is an appropriate place for the spirits. Another reason is also that the west of China is a big expanse of land, and the east is the place of the rising of sun and life. But the spirits are not connected with that aspect in this question, it is more the despair and the poor condition of the spirits which are alluded to here.

Elisabeth Rochat: In the human body the lungs are like a roof or a canopy for all the viscera, especially the heart. They are responsible for all good equilibrium and balance of the *qi*, for calmness, and so on.

The western quarter gives rise to dryness

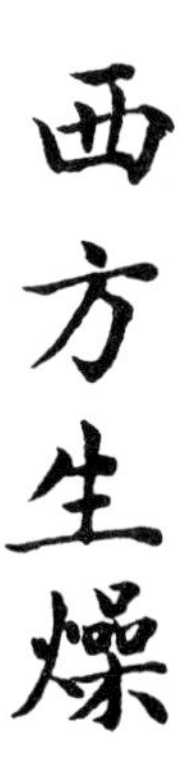

Sheng (生) is the movement of life, the process of life. But how can we connect west and dryness? Father Larre has said that in the west of China there is an area of desert, but what is the explanation of the Chinese people for that? We have to turn to autumn. In autumn the splendid fruits are ripe and full at the beginning, and we need to harvest them, because if they are not harvested they dry out. Autumn is also the period of white frosts, which are a condensation of vapours coming as a consequence of coldness descending onto the earth which is still warm from the summer. In the traditional Chinese calendar the periods corresponding with the season of autumn are the Ending of the Great Heat, White Dew, the Autumn Equinox, Cold Dew and White Frost, and there is a specific accent on the effect of this condensation in the shape of liquids. We find all that in the function of the lung inside the body.

So we can think analogically that the west is the region of condensation and concentration, of vapours and *qi*, and there is no condensation and concentration without a movement of urging and pressing. We find this movement in one of the most important functions of the lung, *qing su* (清 肅), making things such as vapours and *qi* descend in the shape of liquids, by the movement of condensation. It is all in the pressure of the lungs on all the bodily liquids in the trunk. Perhaps through all that we can find a connection between the west and dryness?

Claude Larre: From my own point of view we are not astute enough in our observation of the situation in our own practice. The Chinese say that if you see dew it is a sign of dryness, but we say that if you see dew it is a sign of humidity. But they are right because it proves that the humidity has been taken from the air and is just lying on the surface of the ground. We have to observe the way the Chinese construct their observation of the processes in nature and not just to stick to the result, because the difference between our western minds and the Chinese mind is that the Chinese observe how things develop in themselves, and we are more content with the pure fact of the result. So when they call something dry we are entitled to call it damp, but it is not contradictory. One is one aspect of the dryness in that everything has been taken out, and the other is an aspect of humidity in that since something has been taken out it has to be put somewhere, and it is put on the ground. The fact is that the big region in the west of China is very dry, and that because this is not so in the east it means that for the Chinese, according to their own view of nature, the west is dry. We have to use both ways to understand what they are saying.

Elisabeth Rochat: In pathology we can see that dryness can easily be mixed with cold or warmth. We find that the two seasons before and after autumn are either the warm summer or the cold winter, and there is often a bad equilibrium and unbalanced situation in the dryness, which explains warm dryness and cold dryness. In the main part of China autumn is not the season of rain, and this is seen as the first state of the separation of heaven and earth, because heaven is not giving more to earth in the form of rain.

Dryness gives rise to metal

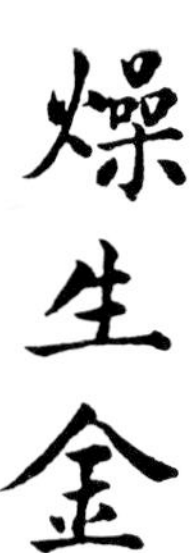

To understand this sentence I think we must connect dryness with this movement of condensation and concentration. As a result of this pressure something goes down into the depths, and if we look at the same movement inside the earth we have metal because metal is simply a condensation and a concentration within the depths of the earth. The ideogram for metal, *jin* (金), depicts the idea of men digging inside soil in order to find metal (Weiger Lesson 14T). You can see at the bottom of the earth two nuggets of gold, so this ideogram, *jin*, means all kinds of metal, or gold. At the top of the ideogram you have the roof of the cave where they are digging. We have something analogous with wood and tree. The same ideogram *mu* (木) has the meaning of wood or a tree, because of all kinds of wood or vegetation the tree is the best example and the most precious with deep roots inside the soil and with the force to rise up towards heaven. Of the metals the most precious is gold, and gold is also the best example because gold is very easy to work although it is very hard.

If you look at the definition of the metal element in all Chinese books you do not find the idea that it is something very hard and strong, rather you find something like the definition in the Book of History, one of the Five Classics:

The property of metal is to obey the hand of the craftsman and to take different shapes.

This is the character of metal, it is both harder than water or wood, but it is also easier to work. For example, water can take any form but cannot keep any form by itself, it just takes the form of its container. It is the same for fire, fire just destroys forms and shapes but it can take its own form. With wood you can cut it, but then it is finished. Yet with metal you can melt it, and melt it again and work it many times. In the same Book of History it says of wood that you can bend it but that it will straighten again, but metal obeys the hand of the craftsman. There is always this dialectic of contraries of the compenetration of life, which is the fundamental point about the logic of China. At the same time this metal is able to make structures and consolidate things. It can keep a form or change it - for example by the action of fire, so for this reason metal is very sensitive to the progress of fire.

In another way metal is the element which has a very brilliant and shining colour, and these qualities are some of the aspects of the colour of the west and of autumn, white. But the metal which has this shining colour is also the instrument of death because from metal you forge arms, swords and so on. This fact is also in the Chinese mind, and by this means metal is also linked with the other aspects of white which is the colour of sunset, of death, of the *po* and of the colour of the bones within the earth after a certain time. So even within the colour of metal we find this double aspect of something shining and of something which can bring death.

Claude Larre: Taking earth as the baseline, a tree has the quality of expanding upwards, going along its own way, but metal has a receding aspect and although it is hard it is also yielding at the same time. It is not like wood which makes its movement by itself, metal is ready to be depressed and oppressed because it is at the end of the process. This is important for the colleges when they teach the five elements, because the teaching should not be restricted to anything other than the process. The process of the elements is used to direct the mind to the pathology, and the *yin yang* effect can be seen in the five elements. One of the best teachings would be to contrast wood and metal according to the Chinese etymology, and then relate that to the condition of the patient and the treatment.

Question: I do not see why, according to that, metal should be shining and wood should be the opposite.

Claude Larre: The fact is that the metal is so pressed and condensed that if you cut it, in the light it shows the ability to reflect. This is not the same as wood. Even though leaves may seem glossy, wood itself is not shiny. If you cut a tree there is just the colour of the tree, but if you cut a piece of metal it will be shiny if there is enough light on it.

Metal gives rise to the acrid taste

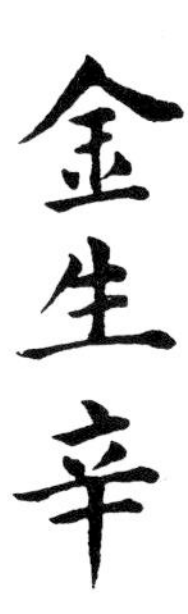

This Chinese idea of taste is not exactly the savour in the

mouth because it is also the internal structure and the more visible and perceptible quality of the essences which compose a particular being. Through the decomposition of the essences you can smell the odour, or you can experience the taste, and you can get an idea of the quality of the essences which constitute the being.

Claude Larre: First we have the smell or the taste which is acrid. That is a perception, which is the same for Chinese and occidentals. But the question is how is it possible that what we taste and what we smell have something in common? If they do have something in common then it must be a quality behind what we perceive, and when something is behind what we perceive we call it a structure. So 'structure' is the word to describe what in one direction is the smell and in the other direction the taste, or in another the colour. The colour, the taste, the smell and the sound have something in common if they are of the western quarter, or the eastern quarter, or wherever. It is not just that because we cannot perceive what lies behind what we perceive it does not exist. The quality of the west can be seen as dryness, or a certain smell, or a certain taste, and the difficulty is that we are not used to this turn of mind. For the Chinese west is not just a division of space but a division of what exists, of life, and there is a quality there which when combined with the other qualities, composes the living being.

If I am able to have a heart, or a liver or kidneys it is just because I am a man and within me these qualities combine to make my *zang*. And when it is not a question of *zang*, when it is a plant, for example, or outside somewhere, what do we call that? It depends. We call it the western region, or the colour blue, or some kind of sound. The Chinese way is very clear, they have divided the unity of the cosmos into five and we call it the five elements or phases. The point is that whenever there is composition or decomposition it is on the level of five. Of course it is true that the perception of individual things does not always correspond exactly to that, for example some things taste acrid but they are not white. But the white the Chinese are talking about is not necessarily the colour white which can be seen. Yet if the white of the Chinese has the same properties as the west or the acrid taste then we can understand what they mean by white.

The trouble is that we are not abstract enough, we want the actual sensation of things. We think we know what white is, but the Chinese answer is that we do not know what white is unless we take our information from Su wen chapter 5. You have to understand that the white alluded to is the white that is seen in the west, and that is different to the white colour seen here on this sheet of paper. But this sheet of paper, being white in the western meaning, is related to the west. It is truly white, but it is not the white you see. Behind what you see there is a structure which when it is seen is white and when it is tasted is acrid. There are two levels and everything goes by five. One level is more abstract, but very concrete! It is only abstract for our sensations. If we can accept the *zang* as we accept them in Chinese medicine why can we not accept the colours and tastes and smells in the Chinese way? The difference between white and west and lung and so on is much less than we think. At one level it is all the same thing. This is very difficult to understand, but it is very logical.

Elisabeth Rochat: The ideogram for acrid is *xin* (辛) (Weiger Lesson 102H). The composition of the ideogram gives the idea of offending a superior. Etymologically the lower part has the meaning of offence, and consequently this ideogram *xin* also has the meaning of what happens after an offence is committed, that is punishment, pain and bitterness. On the physical level it could be a wound or an injury and on the psychological level it could be a painful constriction of the heart. These things are all possible meanings of *xin* as well as acrid. Another meaning of *xin* is as the eighth of the celestial stems, corresponding to west and metal and autumn and so on.

Peter Firebrace: Basically the ten stems are an expansion of the five elements in that you have two stems for each element. So the first and second stems correspond to wood beginning with gallbladder and then liver, and so on round the cycle to fire, small intestine and heart, on to the earth with stomach and spleen, and then on to metal with the colon and then the lung which would be the eighth stem. Following that there would be the stem for the bladder and for the kidneys. You always have the *yang* stem and then the *yin* stem, which is an expansion of the idea of the five elements as a cycle. Instead of having a single element you have the *yang* aspect and then the *yin* aspect of the element. That is the simplest way of seeing the cycle of the ten stems. So here you have the lung which will give way to the stems for water which will be the ninth and tenth stems.

Claude Larre: One may ask how it is possible to go from the five elements to the ten stems? If you think that the virtue of heaven is only *yang*, it is impossible to go to the stems. But this is not true. The virtue of heaven has never been said to be only *yang*, it is *yin* or *yang* depending. This point is not usually taught in the colleges, because teachers are often afraid to take a position on it as they are not sure how it can be. So what Peter said is good, there are five ways to organize the virtue but each of these ways is *yin* or *yang*. So if they are *yin* or *yang*, a system organized by ten is necessary.

To return to what Elisabeth was saying, in autumn there is repression and obedience. People either revolt or submit. It is good for the government if they submit, if they contradict it is not good for the government, but they contradict in an autumn-like fashion. This is very important because in our simple way of thinking about life we say either they obey or they disobey. But this is not true. Either they obey or they disobey according to a certain phase, which in this case is the autumn phase. So, the text is not so difficult to understand if we see that the lungs are constructed from a certain sort of essence, the quality of which is also in autumn or the west, it is the same thing. They have to be in accordance with the position of acrid in the five elements. The text of the Su wen chapter 5 is constructed in a way which expresses the movement of life when organizing all the elements of a living being. So when we come to man we have to come to the *zang*, and the *zang* have to come from somewhere, and they come from acrid because it is a taste and the taste is connected with the essences. The quality for the taste of the west is acrid which is said to produce the lungs, *xin sheng fei* (辛 生 肺).

Elisabeth Rochat: In the same way that Father Larre was describing the nature of acrid in accordance with the movement of metal, of dryness and the west, it is in accordance with this kind of constriction or punishment or pain. But the effect of the acrid taste is diffusion, expansion of *qi* and sometimes humidification. The explanation is the same: only that which is able to concentrate is able to expand. In comparison the acid taste which is connected with the east and spring, corresponds to a movement of expansion, but the effect of the acid taste, according to the Su wen chapter 22, is to collect together. This is exactly the same dialectical explanation.

The acrid taste gives rise to the lung

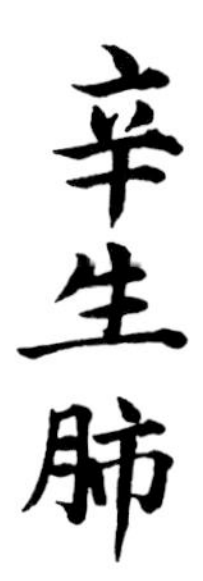

Elisabeth Rochat: How can that be? With 'acrid' we saw that we have to understand the structure of a specific quality of essences which compose a being, or a kind of food, and the essences which are the main component of a thing can first be perceived through the taste and smell. Within my being they can nourish and maintain the movements which express the same quality. In the case of acrid this is found in the lung. If I eat something acrid I am eating something the essences of which are able to nourish and maintain the movement of condensation and concentration within my being. So as a consequence the acrid taste has a special relationship with the lung and constitutes the life of the lung in my body. For this reason we can now understand the sentence 'acrid produces the lung'. Acrid produces the original structure from which the lung can be made, it is like weaving something on a canvas. The lung is not just flesh or tissue, before that it is one of five aspects of the vital movement within an human being.

Claude Larre: Let me recapitulate this. We have a Chinese text which starts with the west. The effect of this is dryness, the effect of dryness is condensation, and the effect of that has to be seen at the level of what is called acrid. Acrid has so many meanings, it is not exactly the taste you have on your tongue but the structure that makes the taste which you experience as acrid. This is only possible when you eat something, so if there is no food there is no taste. And if there is no taste there can be no identification of the food.

The identification of food comes from the fact that there are certain essences present and not others, so taste, food and essences are all the same thing. To be on the same level as something is to be composed of a certain structure which works on the canvas of human life, and in this case at that same level it creates the possibility of being able to have lungs. The lung is not different from acrid which is not different from metal which is not different from dryness which is not different from the west.

You have to follow the line as the Chinese have put it because if you do not do that where will the question of humidity come? Each of these terms can reverse itself, but you are not free to say that dryness is the same thing as humidity, first you have to state how the dryness is produced. Dryness is produced by the west. Then when you have this you can counter the dryness with humidity by the convertibility of terms. What is important is to follow the line, so we arrive here knowing what the difference between acrid and lung is. The difference is that acrid is just acrid in nature and lung is acrid in man, and the development of the lung which is given at birth needs food, food which is of the same characteristic quality and structure as the essences which are on the same canvas. What is the difference between taste and essences? Taste is a more specific feeling we get through eating the food, and essences are less related to food and taste because they are more abstract. When we say essences it is more the philosophy of the thing which is being alluded to.

Question: What word are you translating as essences here?

Claude Larre: Jing (精). If you want to know what essences are you have to take them in the combination of *jing shen* or *jing qi*. It is impossible to give any definition of a single Chinese word! You have to take it inside an expression and if possible to take the expression within a sentence. If you are only working with a single word the context is given by you but if you are working with a sentence the context is given by the text. It is always better to talk Chinese with the Chinese than to talk Chinese with yourself!

Elisabeth Rochat: A definition of essences based on the ideogram could be everything which you can grasp or extract from grains along with the quality of rising vitality signified by the colour green.

The lung gives rise to the skin and body hair

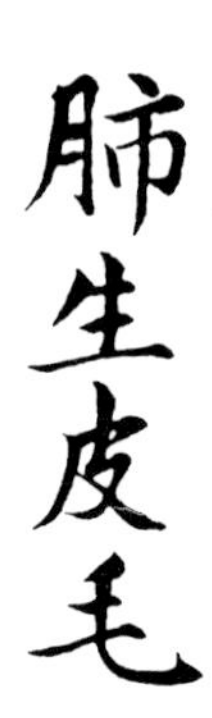

Elisabeth Rochat: Following the same movements and line of thought we can understand skin and body hair as a boundary or limit to the diffusion and expansion of *qi*, and also to the bodily shape. At the skin and body hair we can see the limiting of the loss of vitality which could take place through the pores or the orifices of the skin. The body hair can be understood as the ripening of the 'vegetation' of the body reliant upon the internal vitality, because skin and body hair need the perpetual nourishment of liquid, blood and *qi* etc. Skin and body hair retain the vitality inside and by this means make possible its fructification.

We can see another relationship between lung and skin and body hair in the rhythm of respiration. In the respiration of the skin all the pores and orifices open and close along with the holes of each body hair. Skin and body hair form a whole, unlike, for example, bones and marrow which are produced by the kidneys in the equivalent passage in Su wen chapter 5 and which can appear separately.

Skin and body hair are not exactly a couple, more a whole, forming the superficial area of the body. Skin and body hair appear at the level of human beings in the median between heaven and earth. The west and dryness are also an expression of this movement in heaven or by heaven, and metal and acrid are the expression of this same movement on earth or through earth, with lung, skin and body hair at the level of mankind.

The skin and body hair give rise to the kidneys

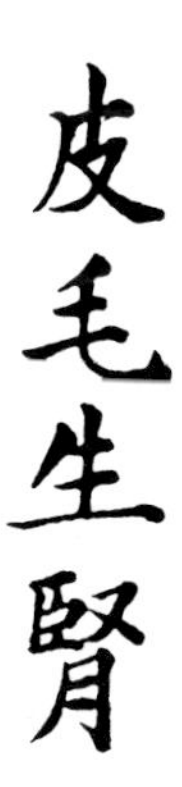

Elisabeth Rochat: Skin and body hair are at the limit of the movement of diffusion and prevent the loss of vitality, for example in the form of sweat. Therefore the skin enables the active and fruitful storage of essences inside the body, especially by the kidneys because the kidneys store essences and allow life to continue at the most internal level. The west, the autumn and so on are the beginning of the return to the *yin* and the increasing of the movement towards the inner depths. It is a descending and concentrating movement, and the beginning of the return to the kidneys which are a basis or foundation. We have here another example of the relationship between metal and water. Metal produces water, and at the internal level the lung condenses the humid vapours and causes the drops of water to descend through the trunk and arrive at the area of the kidneys and bladder.

Claude Larre: The fact is we draw some power from below, and that is the water in the kidneys which is full of fire and water. It is not water as such, but some kind of power which enables us to increase our being. So if we are drawing from below in order to expand it is probably that what is below has been condensed, and for me that is the image of a well. A well is the common place below where all the rain which has fallen and filtered through the ground collects and can be drawn from. If the water we are talking of is the water of life, then this water is what is needed to produce life. So life emerges from the interior of the being, and in order to emerge it has to have been condensed. The condensation is done by the lung, principally through the effect of the skin and body hair, and the water which is then ready to be used is the kidney.

We are not talking of anatomy, we are talking of functions, and when we talk of functions in ourselves they are not separate from functions in the universe. Any function you like has to follow the lines of one of the five classes. If this is condensation it is done through the effect of the lung and for the effect of the kidneys. One is doing an action and the other is taking from that and bringing it further, so the two *zang* are not quoted under the same aspect. This is one of the main difficulties of the text. It took me a long time to understand how it was possible that there could be two *zang* quoted. I thought that when we came to the level of the human being there would be one *zang* and then the text would move on. So we must just keep in mind the process itself, and the images we use are helpful for this.

The lung masters the nose

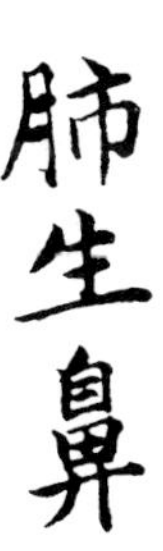

Elisabeth Rochat: This is easy to understand. The nose is the upper orifice by which path the clear *qi* of heaven enters, and the lung is the *zang* connected with the heavenly *qi*, and which is an heaven for the other *zang* and *fu*. Another thing is that it is by the nose that the clear *qi* can descend inside the body, and then within the lung there is a separation between the ascending *qi* for expelling and the descending *qi* going for maintenance of the body and so on.

The lung masters, *zhu* (主), the nose. There is no relation of producing, *sheng* (生), here. The important thing is not that the lung can produce an orifice but that in the construction and structure of the body it is the lord or sovereign over its vassal, the nose. Like a vassal it must observe the boundaries in order to see whether perverse barbarians are approaching, and it too is observed. If the nose is blocked or something perhaps the lungs are not in a good state, because using this analogy we can get an idea of the lord from his vassal and vice versa.

Claude Larre: Usually when we talk of a master we feel that the master is more important than the servant, but that is not true because if the master no longer takes care of the servant there is no more servant. The master is the master and the servant is the servant, and when you accept that you can see things from the other side and say I should be a good master in order to keep my servant. And the servant says I have a job and I should stick to it because at this time it is not so easy to find a good master. So the lung and the nose are also related to each other in this way. This is very important because some of us may think that since the lung is a *zang* and the nose is just an orifice the *zang* is more precious than the orifice. But that is not true. I refer you to Zhuang zi chapter 2. Inside the body everything is in circulation and there is also a hierarchy with the *zang* at a high level. But the Chinese way of feeling that high level is that it has to pretend to be more or less at the service of the lower level. One level is just facing the other. In the Chinese way one is not more important than the other.

The character *zhu* (主) appears in the seventh position in this series of sentences. Up to this point it has been *sheng* (生) which has been used to describe the relationship between the two qualities, but after these first six statements you have the addition of another one with *zhu* as the verb. This brings you to the level of seven, the level of life. But the level of life relies on the six relations which appear before it. So here we can understand how the Chinese play with numbers.

SU WEN CHAPTER 8
THE LUNG AS MINISTER AND CHANCELLOR

The lung has the charge of minister and chancellor.
Thus the regulation of the relays for animation is brought about.

Elisabeth Rochat: In Su wen chapter 8 the lung comes in second position immediately after the presentation of the heart. The heart is the lord and master and from him come all the radiance and illumination of the spirits. Just after the heart, the lord and sovereign, comes the lung like a minister and chancellor, *xiang fu* (相 傅). *Fu* (傅) does not exactly mean chancellor but it is difficult to translate. The impression of *xiang fu* is of a person who helps his master. The lung is situated in the upper part of the trunk just beside the heart, the lord, so the lung protects, covers and envelopes it. The lung is very close to the heart just as the chancellor is very close to the lord.

The result of having this charge of being minister and chancellor is that:

Thus the regulation of the relays for animation, zhi jie chu (治 節 出) *is brought about.*

The 'regulation' is the ideogram *zhi* (治). It is a way of governing. The same ideogram is used meaning to treat or to cure, or to know how to manage a situation. In the case of a government you have to know how to govern the country, in the case of a body you have to know how to conduct your life or how to cure the vitality in another individual. These seem different meanings in our vocabulary, but in reality they are the same thing. The ideogram *jie* (節) means relays, it has the bamboo radical (no.118). In this image all the relays of and for animation are found because animation always proceeds and progresses by relays. Relays are just different stages, and life or vitality proceeds by stages, never by a straight line. Animation needs relays just as bamboo needs knots in its structure. All life is articulations, articulations between *yin* and *yang*, between the five elements or between the twelve meridians. In special contexts *jie* can also mean acupuncture points because these can be seen as articulations in the animation. Articulations can be the stages of development in the *qi* of the life of a person, and as acupuncture points these are the relays of animation and the stages of circulation of each quality of *qi*.

How and why is the lung minister and chancellor? How and why can he regulate all these relays of animation? He stands beside the heart, and he masters the *qi*. In mastering the *qi* he can propagate and diffuse all kinds of *yin* and *yang qi* and send it into circulation right up to the skin and body hair. You know that from the upper heater and the sea of *qi* in the middle of the chest, nutritive and defensive *qi* is sent everywhere in the body. Classical commentaries emphasize the fact that it is through the lung that *yin* and *yang qi* are sent forth and mastered. Another aspect of this is that because the lung masters the *qi* and each morning receives the carriers of the network of animation, all the *mo* or *mai*, at the court audience, it can regulate them and put them into good balance again. And the regulation by the lung is done through all the relays of animation.

Another aspect of this is respiration, either by the nose or by the skin. Respiration is the rhythm of good circulation given to the *qi* of the body. This is due to the lung.

Also, when the heart is acting as the master of blood and

the whole network of animation, he is acting in a couple with the lung which is mastering *qi*. The circulation and compenetration of blood and *qi* all takes place between heart and lung. It is like a country which is well governed by a Lord and his Minister who have a good understanding.

Claude Larre: I would just like to make some sort of correlation between what was said previously and what has been said now. When we talked of Su wen chapter 2 it was just to show the balance of *yin* and *yang*, because chapter 2 is about that. It describes how the *qi* of a man follows the sway of *yin* and *yang* in nature. In chapter 5 we saw that the organization of life was the topic, and that organization has to be made by five. Here in chapter 8 it is no longer a question of the organization of the lung as such. The chapter asks how all of that plays its role in the government of life. All the terminology is based on the analogy of the body with the government of a state, so in first place some lordship has to be present to control everything. But the more you control the less you are visibly acting, because the more you interfere the less things go as they should go! If you let things go unchecked, there will be no control over the activity of the government, so there must be a minister somewhere in order to carry out the will and to bear the responsibility of the head of state. This is the role of the lung as minister and chancellor.

The difference we are making between minister and chancellor is very refined, and is taken from the Chinese text. If we say minister we are insisting that he is the head of all the other ministers, while if we say chancellor we are talking of administration at large. Every order or nomination given has to be stamped by some authority so that the subjects can recognize that this pertains to the life of the country, or in the case of the lung, the life of the body. The lung needs to be close to the heart in order to represent the active part of the heart.

As far as the question of knots or relays, *jie* (節), is concerned, I would say that it is quite normal for there to be regular moves in life if man is just a result of the activity of heaven and earth. The regular moves are a rhythm, and we know that the *tian yun* (天 湞), the large circulations of the influence of heaven which make life in the universe, have a corresponding factor in our own life. We know that if there is a rhythm in the virtue of heaven, the same rhythm and virtue is exerting itself in our own life. But heaven itself does not take care of the rhythm in us because it is so high and powerful, instead its deputy and minister the lung does. The lung makes the will of heaven consistent in our own bodily life. So if the *jie* are seen more as bony articulations it is just because heaven is expressing its own presence through earth, and our earthly aspect is more in the direction of visible flesh and bones. But it takes the same *qi* to make bones or flesh or tissues or to make the body go through some rhythm. You see more if it is bones or flesh and you see less if it is respiration, but behind it all is the fact that the virtue of heaven has to express itself. In itself the virtue of heaven is not visible, but we are here in order to make it visible. This is why they use *jie* to refer to the twenty-four different articulations in the calendar's weather, and why they do the same thing for the rhythm of life. Articulations also have to be in certain places, and if there are places then perhaps they may also be touched by a needle!

Elisabeth Rochat: Father Larre just mentioned the use of *jie* as being like an articulation of time or weather. During the year there are twenty-four divisions of time which are called the knots of *qi*, *jie qi* (節 氣), or climatic periods. Each one is fifteen days. The meaning of this is that time, like everything else, is a quality of *qi*, and each fifteen days the quality changes in a perceptible way. Fifteen is five multiplied by three, five is a small number of days perhaps related to the five elements, and three is the number of *qi*. In five days you could not really feel the difference, but in fifteen days you can feel something different. The twenty-four periods of the year set the rhythm of social life because each period had a name which indicated the work of the labourer in the fields, and all the feasts.

Classical Chinese texts just after the Nei jing said that the lung had twenty-four 'holes', or hollows, or perhaps the alveoli. The ideogram is *kong* (空), which is something like a void. The lung ensures and sums up all the articulations of *qi* in space and time, and if they are able to do that their internal structure must reflect it. It is impossible in the Chinese mind that a thing can have a function and not be the natural structure for that function. If the lung is able to master and regulate all the relays of animation in space and time it must therefore have twenty-four holes or voids in its structure to do that.

Certain texts more recent than the Nei jing but prior to the nineteenth century say that the lung is the first bodily structure to be finished because when a baby is born he is able to cry and breathe. The lung is also said to be like the trunk of life for mankind. In one particular text it then says that the liver comes next when the baby opens its eyes, then the spleen is finished completely when the baby is able to eat, and the heart when the baby is able to laugh and speak, giving out noises which are not just cries, and the kidneys when the baby can stand up firmly. And a man is completely finished when he reaches his normal height and has his wisdom teeth. In the same text it says that at the end of life the lung is the last to wear out because if the *qi* is not interrupted and respiration continues you are not dead. But all this is not in the oldest texts!

This function of the lung as a minister and helper to the heart can also be seen in Ling shu chapter 36.

SU WEN CHAPTER 9

The lung is the trunk in which the qi is rooted.
It is the residence of the po.
Its flourishing aspect is in the body hair.
The power of its fullness is in the skin.
It is the tai yin within the yang.
It is in free communication with the qi of autumn.

Elisabeth Rochat: We can see several different aspects here. First of all the lung in relationships with *qi*, with the *po* (魄), and with the skin, and afterwards the relationship with heaven and the clear *qi* of heaven and the movement of expansion. In Su wen chapter 62 it says that the lungs store *qi*. Ling shu chapter 8 says the same thing. In Su wen chapter 9 each of the five *zang* are presented as a trunk of vital elements in the human body. The heart goes first which is like the trunk of life itself. Next comes the lung which is 'the trunk in which the *qi* is rooted', *ben* (本).

Then follows the kidneys which are like the trunk of all kinds of storage, hibernation and so on, and the liver which is like the trunk from which activity can stop. Finally comes the spleen, along with the five *fu* (附) for transformation, which is like the trunk for all kinds of granaries, barns and so on. So you can see the heart and lung are in a special position with a particular function for each. This means that all the *qi* in the body coming from every activity and each *zang* and *fu* is under the overlord lung, which gives to it all that is essential for life, for example a good rhythm, regulation and the relays of animation. The lung gives all *qi* the possibility of expressing itself in a good way.

'The lung is the residence, *chu* (處), of the *po* (魄)'. It is a place from which the *po* can disperse their activity. We saw the *po* in Ling shu chapter 8 where they are linked with the lung.

Claude Larre: When we say 'place' or 'residence' we have to remember that the lung is an active facet of life, so if there is a place there must be a special power because in Chinese you never talk of a place without talking of the power related to that place. A place is therefore a place from which you can do something. So just as the place of the heart is related to the *shen* (神) so the lung is related to the *po*. But the way these two things are presented is not exactly the same because the character used to describe the relationship of heart to *shen* is *bian* (變), change, because we know that the *shen* are free to come and go and have a more airy movement. The *po* do not change, they are related to earth while the *shen* are related to heaven.

Elisabeth Rochat: In the ideogram for *po* (魄) on the left side there is the colour white, *bai* (白). The other part is a spirit of earth, *gui* (鬼). *Shen* are spirits of heaven and the *gui* are spirits of earth. *Hun* (魂) and *po* (魄) both have this same radical no.194. In *hun* it is put together with the image of clouds (云), which are just the gathering up in heaven of the vapour rising from earth. In *po* it is put together with white (白), the colour of sunset. The *po* are linked with a descending movement and with essences. In human life the *po* have all vital movement, perception and instinctive movement under their authority. But since the lung store the *qi*, why are they also linked with the essences and downward movement, all things contrary to *qi*, via these spirits? And why are the *hun*, which are exactly like *qi* in their expanding and rising up movements linked with the liver which stores blood. The answer is always the same. If you want to have compenetration it has to be made between two complimentary things not two similar things. So if the lung stores and masters *qi* it is necessary that the *po* be linked with them because they can form a *yinyang* couple. The *po*, linked with essences, can grasp and be grasped by *qi*.

Question: You said *po* are linked with essences, could you say something more about that?

Elizabeth Rochat: This is mentioned in Ling shu chapter 8 where there is a description of *jing* (精), *shen* (神), *hun* (魂) and *po* (魄). The definition of the *hun* is that they can come and go with the *shen* and the definition of the *po* is that they can go out and come in again in association with the *jing*. In all old Chinese texts we find the *hun* in association with spirits and *po* with essences. Sometimes we can see that *hun* are like the soul of *qi* and *po* are like the soul of essences, or *hun* like the *yang* aspect of spirits and *po* like the *yin* aspect.

In the sentence where the *po* 'go out and come in in association with the essences', we find once again the idea of the rhythm of life. The ideograms to go out, *chu* (出), and to come in, *ru* (入), are vast in their meanings. The first going out is birth and the last coming in is death, it is just an appearance and disappearance with a form, a shape and a body in between forming individual life. Another possible meaning could be respiration, because in that process air is coming in and going out, and it is linked with the lung. There is also the input of food and the expelling of waste. We can also have in mind the infinite number of comings in and goings out through the pores, and all the interactions of *qi*. All reactions, especially instinctive reactions, are under the authority of the *po*.

In this coming in and going out there is not much freedom, it is very strict. Respiration, birth and death and all kinds of reaction are not the expression of someone's freedom. The important thing in goings out and comings in at every level is the grasping of elements of vitality in the form of essences, for example through respiration, or digestion or through the whole grasping of perception. The natural relationship of *po* is with the movement of association, for the *hun* it is the movement of following. The *hun* follow the spirits and the *po* are in association with the essences. The essences are the expression of the power of descending and concentration and earth. After death the essences are no longer linked with the *qi* and are free to follow their own natural movement, so they return to the lower part and to earth, in particular through the lower orifices. Spirits, especially the *po*, need doors to go out of, even if they are very fine and subtle doors. Pores are doors and orifices are doors, and even your heart is a door, although it is not a material one. The 'gate of *po*' is the anus, and throughout your life the *po* pass through that door in the form of waste. One ideogram for waste (粕) is made up with white and a grain of cereal. When you eat, all the vitality that you can grasp, digest and incorporate into your being is the *jing*, the essences, and all the other part, which is waste, goes out of you via the anus. This is the descending part of alimentation. In death there is only the separation of elements which in compenetration made life. When the knot of life is untied, the *po* return to earth.

Question: In relation to chapter 9 what is the significance of number nine?

Claude Larre: This is still a question for me! Usually if nine comes after eight it proves that nine is the expression of a more complex activity than what is expressed by eight. So, because eight and nine are quite far from the beginning, but quite near when compared with eighty-one, it proves that in presenting life and the interconnection of the different elements we have been distinguishing, eight and nine are very close to each other. But perhaps we will see how eight is made more clearly when we see nine. One chapter usually relies on the preceding chapter if the series of chapters is taken at the low numbers, from about one to twelve. That would not be true for the others because it is too complicated to enter the field of interpretation. But it would be valuable to register all the information given in chapter 9 about lung and liver and so on, because some words would be the same and some would be different and this would give the specificity of one *zang* in relation to another. If the same Chinese word is used for different things this tells us something. The text is so precise that when it is different there is a meaning and when it is similar it proves that the things are on the same level.

Coming back to the question of roots, as in chapter 9: 'The lung is the trunk in which the *qi* is rooted'. When we say rooted, if in our mind it is just the place where things are, that is not enough. The meaning of *ben* (本) is to be attached to the place where things are made. Something is said to be rooted exactly where it stems from, so just as in gardening, you must take care of the roots above everything.

Its flourishing aspect is in the body hair
The power of its fullness is in the skin

Elisabeth Rochat: We saw this before, that the expression of the fullness of the power of the lung, through the *qi* and circulation is perceptible through the good state of the skin and good defence at that level. This is an easy connection with the defensive *qi* which is passed into circulation through the impulse of the lung, even if it is coming from the lower heater and ascending through the middle heater to reach the upper heater. The nutritive *qi* also circulates in the meridians through the impulse of the lung, and *tai yin* (太陰), the lung meridian, opens the circulation of the twelve meridians. Also, it is particularly through *yang qi*, and to a lesser extent, defensive *qi*, that the lung can give a good rhythm to the opening and closing which takes place at the level of the skin.

It is the tai yin within the yang

This is the maximum power of *yin*, so why is it not connected with winter and the kidneys? I think it is because *tai yin* is the *yin* which can show magnificent effects, in the shape of fruits and harvest, of the produce of the earth, so in this way it is the autumn and the *zang* linked with autumn which can be a *tai yin* more than the *zang* linked with winter which is the imperceptible power of life through *yin* just showing the separation and the bareness. Winter is the *yin* in its *shao* (少) aspect, while from this perspective autumn is the *yin* in its magnificence. But in other non-medical texts such as the Book of Changes you find autumn as the beginning of *yin* in *shao yin*, and *tai yin* as the maximum *yin* power in winter. According to commentaries, when the text says: 'It is the *tai yin* within the *yang*', the *yang* is referring to the part of the trunk above the diaphragm, which is the *yang* part and houses the heart and lung. Chapter 9 also calls the heart the *tai yang* within the *yang*.

It is in free communication with the qi of autumn

We saw this previously, that the same quality of *qi* and movement of autumn can be found in a human being in the lung. Actually, we should say that the same quality of *qi* and movement of autumn *are* the lung in a human body, because there is no lung if there is not this movement and quality of *qi*.

Claude Larre: The invisible function is always more telling than the physical anatomy of an organ. The primary conception of the text is the function, and that is why they talk of *tai yin* and so on. If they are talking of the *yin* and *yang* aspects it proves they are more concerned with the way that life is functioning, and only after that comes a consideration of the physical, objective, sensible, concrete reality which you can cut out and replace. It is the void, *kong* (空), the invisible and the *yin* and *yang* aspects which are the concern of the text. So once again we have to warn people not to start from their pre-conceived ideas of what a heart or lung is and then try to fix that from the text, we must just follow what is given. We must interpret Su wen chapter 10 in the same way:

The lung: its reunion is in the skin

The meaning of this is that the movement which is the lung inside the body, is the skin on the exterior of the body at the level of the materialized structure of the body. For this reason the skin and the lung are interlinked by this *he* (呵), this conjunction of *qi*. So if this movement of life is disturbed at the level of the skin there can easily be a reaction at the level of the lung because they are an harmonic.

THE LUNG AS A CANOPY

Elisabeth Rochat: In various chapters of the Nei jing the lung is said to be like a roof or canopy for the heart and the other *zang* and *fu*, for example in Ling shu chapter 29 it says:

The lung is like a canopy for the five zang and the six fu

and in Su wen chapter 46 it says:

The lung is a canopy for the zang

Consequently when the *qi* of the lung is increasing its power all the network of animation is great and large, but if the *qi* of the lung is too strong and powerful then the network of animation and therefore the pulses are too strong too, and the person is unable to lie down quietly. The meaning is that if the lung is like a canopy, a roof or an heaven, it has to be very regular, and possessing a good rhythm, and if the *qi* is too powerful it acts like a countercurrent because it goes too strongly, is excessive and rises up too much, so you find the rhythm of animation is disturbed and the person will be panting.

What is a canopy? It is not simply a roof or a little piece of tissue or material over a bed or a throne, or something like an umbrella extended over an important person. This kind of canopy has to attract a good influx from on high, and to transmit that to the person below. In this case, if the lung is called a canopy for the heart and the other *zang* and *fu*, it is because it is in charge of attracting the influence of heaven and translating it to the others, particularly through the network of animation, essences, *qi* and so on. Therefore, if the natural current is too strong or too weak through excess or deficiency of power, there will be a general malaise as exampled in Su wen chapter 46.

In Su wen chapter 44 there is another presentation:

The lung is called the leader of the zang

The leader here does not mean the same as it does when we say the heart is the lord and sovereign, the leader is just the one who is at the head or the front of the march. This chapter speaks about illnesses connected with *wei* (痿) syndrome. *Wei* syndrome can attack each *zang* but generally speaking it is under the mastership of the lung because this kind of impotence can cause a lessening in the distribution of the lung and in particular of the liquids of the lung and the liquids in all parts of the body by means of the impulse of *qi*. If the lung receives any kind of dryness or warmth it burns and is unable to distribute, or participate in the distribution of *qi* or the liquids which are carried by the *qi* to the four limbs.

Claude Larre: A good analogy is the abbot in a temple. The temple has several buildings, with the rear part higher than the others and having a roof with a sort of canopy featuring a couple of dragons perhaps, and with a courtyard inside, a *yuan* (院). The abbot who presides over all this complex is the *yuan zhang* (院 長), he is the principal, and his authority is exerted for the good of all the people who are inside. He has the position of elder among the others who are brothers, he leads the way.

Elisabeth: Rochat: We have another quotation in Su wen chapter 18 which asks what is really authentic in the storing or the power of the *zang*? It says that when storage is carried out in the highest position it is done through the lung, and it causes defensive and nutritive *qi* to circulate, and the *yin* and *yang*. This means that inside the body by means of the five *zang* or through the five ways to actively store essences, we see the releasing of *qi* at the heart of life.

For the heart there is the possibility of being in free communication, for the spleen it is the possibility to make good irrigation, and for the lung it is to ensure the highest position, in other words to be in the heights like the *qi* of heaven, and to be the highest among the *zang*. The purpose of this is to make defensive and nutritive *qi* circulate well, because in the highest position the lung has the quality of the *qi* of heaven which makes things circulate. The lung has the charge of being minister and chancellor, and the minister and chancellor can establish and maintain harmony between all parts of the country or organism, and can propagate *qi* and the will of the lord and sovereign through *qi*.

Here we have a connection with the sea of *qi*, which is not the lung but is connected with it because its location is between the two lobes of the lung. The ancient texts say that the lung is just a single *zang*, but since the Nan jing they also say that it is divided into two parts.

THE LUNG AND THE QI

Elisabeth Rochat: In the last part of Su wen chapter 5 different qualities of *qi* are placed in connection with various *zang* and *fu*. For the lung it says that the *qi* of heaven is in free communication with or through it. The *qi* of heaven is clear, *qing* (清), and the *qi* of the lung has to be clear and fresh, as is said in Su wen chapter 2 for instance. It also says that the lung, being like a roof or canopy, is also like an heaven for the other *zang* and *fu*. In old texts of around the sixth and seventh centuries the lung is referred to as the heaven within the body. So if the lung is a canopy, a leader and an heaven, it has exactly the same movement as heaven itself, in other words to distribute influence, to put into movement, to give impulse to circulation and propagation, and also to make rain descend to earth. All these functions are found within the lung itself in its movement of expansion, diffusion and distribution of influx not only to the skin but to the *zang* and *fu* and the heart. And at the same time the lung causes liquids to descend.

The connection with heaven is well explained and expounded in Ling shu chapter 78, which is a chapter where the meaning of each number is given in accordance with medical theory and the parts of the human body. At the beginning is one, which is heaven, and heaven is *yang*, and among the *zang* it is the lung which corresponds with heaven because the lung is the canopy of the five *zang* and six *fu*. Skin is in reunion, *he* (合), with the lung, and the skin is the *yang* part of man because it is at the surface and exterior.

In Ling shu chapter 40 you can find differentiated everything that is clear and unclear in the human body. The clear *qi* comes to the lung through the *qi* of respiration, which is clear in contrast to the *qi* of alimentation. Clear, *qing* (清), and unclear, *zhuo* (濁), never designate anything precise but only a movement, or a tendency. It is exactly like *yin* or *yang*, they are always and only understandable in context, and with respiration and alimentation one is clear and one is unclear in comparison to the other. But in another context some parts of alimentation are clear and some are unclear. For example, the essences which are extracted at the level of the middle heater and which can be incorporated by the person are clear, and they can rise up to the upper heater. The five *zang* receive essences in the shape of the five tastes which they work on to release *qi* which eventually all returns to the lung. You also know that the junction of the clear from respiration and the clear from alimentation at the level of the upper heater is the sea of *qi* and the ancestral *qi*, *zong qi* (宗 氣). *Zong qi* has a very special function for respiration because it is through its activity that man can inhale and exhale.

Another characteristic of clear *qi* is that it has a special affinity with all voids, holes and orifices, which brings us back to the structure of the lung and the orifices on the skin and the whole rhythm of opening and closing. From this perspective, therefore, the lung is allowed to receive all that is clear, both directly from heaven and from alimentation. The circulation through the meridians, the beating of the heart and the movement of respiration depend on this. We can also mention at this point the special trajectory of *xu li* (虛 里), the great *luo* (絡) of the stomach, because it is a connection between the diaphragm and the upper heater where it passes through the lung like a network of ramifications and branchings in order to distribute influx. Afterwards it goes out under the left breast, which is the beating of the heart.

In order to finish looking at the connection of the lung with all kinds of *qi* there is a quotation from Ling shu chapter 56:

Grains come into the stomach, and afterwards there is jing wei (精 微).

This is the intermediate state of the essences which compose the alimentation and the essences which compose our life. Food has to be decomposed in order to become the pattern of our own vitality, but the decomposition must not injure the vitality of the essences. After the decomposition the essences can be recomposed through the *zang* and the special activity of the kidneys. The quotation continues:

The jing wei first springs out at the middle and upper heaters in order to water the five zang. This springing out is made in two ways, by nutrition and defence.

Through this you can see the movement of communication of the most subtle essences of alimentation with the middle and upper heaters, and then the differentiation of the two circulations of nutrition and defence. The middle heater gives the elements of composition realized in nutritive and defensive *qi*, the upper heater gives the movement of propagation and distribution.

The great qi beating and accumulating in the middle of the chest is called the sea of qi, and it goes and spreads out through the lung, and afterwards it follows the pharynx.

This shows the connection of this great *qi*, which is the ancestral *qi*, with the lung. It is through the activity of the lung that the connection between the essences of alimentation and respiration can be in activity everywhere in the body giving the movement of life. So if the *zong qi* is responsible for the going out and coming in of respiration and for the beating of the heart, then we can see again this idea of rhythm everywhere.

In Ling shu chapter 62 it says:

The qi of the stomach rises and flows out to the lung, and afterwards it goes to the orifices of the head, the face and the brain.

So there is no circulation of the *qi* of the middle heater if not by the force of the lung.

You can see the relationship of the lung with defensive *qi* at the level of the skin and body hair, which ensures warmth and good irrigation of the superficial flesh and skin amongst other aspects. The circulation of nutritive *qi* also begins through the lung meridian, and afterwards goes through the twelve meridians and *du mai* (督 脈) and *ren mai* (任 脈) before returning to the middle of the lung from where it goes into the body with the *tai yin* (太 陰) and the *yang ming* (陽 明).

Question: When you said that in Ling shu chapter 62 the *qi* of the stomach rises up to the lung, was that referring to the relation of the nutrition with *ying qi*, because usually it is the spleen energy which is said to rise up?

Elisabeth Rochat: In this case it is in relation to *wei qi* (衛 氣), defensive *qi*, because it is to do with this movement of rising up and threading through. *Tai yin* (太 陰) is also first in the circulation of nutritive *qi*, and Ling shu chapter 18 says that *tai yin* masters the interior, because the nutritive *qi*, which first goes to *tai yin* is for the maintenance of the interior.

Question: Are the texts clear about the specific pathways of *wei qi*, or do they just say it is more superficial in the day time and deeper at night?

Elisabeth Rochat: Well, when you first wake you do not have enough sensation to perceive small details, but when you are wide awake you have all the subtlety of perception, and all this is in relation to the defensive *qi*.

Claude Larre: To be defensive you have to be on the alert, and to be on the alert you have to use all your senses, and to do that you have to have enough *qi*.

Question: But if the *wei qi* flows deeper into the *zang* at night that does not seem very defensive!

Claude Larre: That is the reason why you lock your house, you lock your door, and you lock yourself in your bed and close your eyes. Then, if you feel protected, you sleep. It is a question of heart, because if you feel safe the guard can come inside the palace, but if you feel the enemy is outside even if it is night you put sentries on the walls and guards everywhere.

Elisabeth Rochat: It is part of the function of *wei qi* to conserve the well-balanced equilibrium between the *zang*, so it is not just the role of nutrition to support this. Defence and nutrition are not really separable.

Question: Is there any significance in the link between seven and the *po* (魄)?

Claude Larre: Elisabeth has not been able to find any particular teaching giving one specific task to one *po* as distinct from another *po*, so it is better to consider the number seven as the telling feature. We know that seven is the level where something emerged from the six relations, and that this describes the conditions of life. When someone lives in an human body, this body opens to the outside world through the seven orifices, and in order to take care of these seven orifices it is necessary that the *qi* of the orifices is organised. This is done by the *po*.

We know that the *hun* (魂) and the *po* (魄) are characteristics of human life at the level which is under the spirits of heaven and the spirits of earth. More precisely heaven gives life, and when earth and heaven join together there is human life. The joining together of heaven's power and earth's obedience is made through the essences, but there are no essences in human life except through the *shen* (神). The *jing shen* (精 神) are really the way to describe life at the highest level. But under the *shen* comes the *hun* and under the *jing* comes the *po*. The associations of *jing shen* (精 神), *hun po* (魂 魄), *xue qi* (血 氣) and all the others represent different views of this marvellous product of the conjunction of heaven and earth which we call a human being. And if we recognize seven orifices it is normal to recognize seven *po* which together with the three *hun* give the number ten as the mark of the human species. This is referred to in Lao zi chapter 10, which is older than the Nei jing.

The fact that this is chapter 10 gives us one more reason to think that the symbolism of the numbers has been devised in order to show the correlation between three and seven and *hun* and *po.* Rather on the same level we say that the concentration of the virtue of heaven is in the sun, and the number of the sun is ten, and if in mankind there is some kind of supernatural light there is the power of the sun working in that person, which at the highest level we call the spiritual. From that view, the number of the sun, the number of mankind, and the addition of the three *hun* and the seven *po* are joined in the number ten. This gives the inner foundation for having seven *po* even if we are not able to make a distinction between their separate offices.

Elisabeth Rochat: Let us look at the situation where the heart is disturbed by grief, *bei* (悲), which is linked with the lung. Su wen chapter 39 says when a man is full of grief the system of connection which is natural to the heart is tight. This is a special network of connection by which the heart can be in free communication with the viscera called *xin xi* 心 系). By means of this the heart can give the other *zang* the influx of the spirits. If a man is full of grief this *xin xi* is not well relaxed but is tight, *ji* (急). In this state the lung is affected because the lung masters *qi* and receives all *qi* and all networks of animation, and if the *xin xi* is too tight there will be a blockage. The lung will rise up and the free circulation of the *qi* of the upper heater which is normally ensured by the lung falls into a bad state, and the warmth which comes from the blockage can destroy the *qi*.

In Ling shu chapter 36 we can see the same situation where the heart is sad and full of grief and the *xin xi* is tight, *ji* (急). Because of this the lung rises upwards and the eyes overflow with liquid, tears. If the bodily liquids can only circulate with the movement of *qi*, and if because of grief this *qi* is moving in a countercurrent, then the *qi* rises to the upper parts of the body and to the upper orifices and it carries the liquids with them. And this movement can even carry the liquids outside of the body.

This chapter of the Ling shu says the lung cannot always remain in a high position, but must descend again, and for this reason you will get different kinds of coughing or sobbing accompanied by tears falling. So this is a pathological link between heart and lung. If the bodily liquids go upwards when moving countercurrent, then the normal current is for them to go downwards through the lung. This is also explained in Su wen chapter 21.

THE LUNG AND QI IN SU WEN CHAPTER 21

Elisabeth Rochat: Su wen chapter 21 explains the process of the assimilation of solid and liquid food. By solid and liquid we do not have to understand something actually solid or liquid. Rather, we need to see that what is able to restore and maintain human vitality when it is solid is *yang* and its *qi* is strong and hard, and when it is liquid it is able to restore and maintain the *yin*. Do not take the solid and liquid too literally, it is the effect which is important. The character for food in general or solid food in particular is *shi* (食), and for liquid food it is *yin* (飲). Su wen chapter 21 says the liquid food enters the stomach, and after that (it is not in the text but we can imagine it) the stomach and the middle heater transform and digest it and make *jing wei* (精微). Then there is propagation, in the manner of an overflowing, and diffusion of the essences and *qi* because the stomach is a great sea for all essences and *qi*. It is by means of digestion that all renewal of essences and *qi* inside the body is possible, and the *yin* part of the body can thus be restored.

The first movement of these essences and *qi* is ascending and moving up, so they go to the spleen where the essences are diffused and return to the lung.

By means of the lung all waterways and waterings are in

free circulation and well regulated. The descending movement of the lung transports the liquids to the bladder. The essences of water (which represent the vitality of the liquid power of the organism) are diffused in the four directions.

So the movement is very simple: food enters the stomach from where part of it descends to the intestines, and the other part, the essences, goes to the spleen in a movement of overflowing, and from there it goes to the lung which regulates all the waterways, and then downwards by the lung's movement to the bladder. So the lung has exactly the same place as heaven in the schema since this overflowing is a kind of vaporization. Liquids can be humid vapours and here they are like clouds which let rain fall, just as the essences fall to the bladder in liquid form.

There is an expression *qing su* (清 肅), which appears after the time of the Nei jing, that presents this function of the lung in having only clear *qi* which can exert pressure and make vapours or *qi* or liquids descend. *Qing* (清) means clear and pure and fresh. We know that any warmth in the lung means the destruction of *qi* and the countercurrent movement of liquids, so it is especially important that in autumn and in the lung that the *qi* is always clear and fresh. *Su* (肅) means to be respectful, which suggests a bowing motion. In China it is very impolite to have your head higher than that of the man who is your superior! To be respected you have to exert some sort of pressure or force on people, and this is like the movement of autumn, it has a repressive effect. *Su* implies a descending movement. If you remember in Ling shu chapter 18 the upper heater was described as resembling a mist, and in the lung there is the movement for the circulation of *qi* and liquids. In some commentaries *qi* is said to be the mother of water because without *qi* it is impossible to have water or liquids or to have them circulate. This is exactly like heaven, where clouds sometimes circulate slowly or fast, or sometimes let rain fall. The lung is like a turning place for the progress of liquids in the trunk, when the *qi*, loaded with humidity or dampness arrive at this canopy or roof, it has to return to the earth below.

If we return to the beginning of chapter 21 we have another scheme concerning the progress of solid foods:

The qi of solid food enters the stomach, the essences are diffused towards the liver and (by the effect of the function of the liver these essences) ...impregnate muscles with qi.

This is hard to translate, but what it means is that the *qi* of solid food, after the operation of transformation enters the stomach. Then, the essences which are produced go to the liver, from where they impregnate all muscles with *qi*. After this the text goes on that the unclear *qi* from the solid food inside the stomach returns to the heart. We saw this morning that unclear *qi* can represent *qi* coming from the digestion of food in contrast to *qi* from respiration. So in this case unclear *qi* can mean *qi* from digestion. The *qi* from the stomach going to the heart rises up so it is easy to see that it is unclear only because it is coming from digestion, otherwise they would not be able to rise upwards.

Claude Larre: We know the distinction between *yin* and *yang*, but we know there is *yin* of *yin* and *yang* of *yin* and so on. It is the same here, when you say clear or unclear it depends at what level you are talking. The first division is between food and respiration, but inside the food and inside the respiration you make another division of clear and unclear.

Elisabeth Rochat: From the heart the essences impregnate the network of animation, *mai* (脈). This might be in the form of blood for example, because *mai* is also in charge of the network of blood, and of all the nutritive essences for the body and so on. All these things circulate in the *mai* under the domination of the heart, so just as the liver masters the muscles, the heart masters the *mai*. Therefore you can see that the *qi* of solid food restores the activity of the muscles and the network of animation in the human body through the dialectic of essences and *qi* and through the two male *zang*, the liver and the heart.

After that the *qi* of all the network of animation circulates and propagates through all the meridians, and the *qi* of all the meridians returns to the lung. This is important because we can see that the lung is the only *zang* which is involved in the processing of solid food and liquid food. It is at this point in the text in Su wen chapter 21 that we have the famous sentence:

The lung receives the 100 mai in morning audience.

The lung carries essences to the skin and body hair, moving with this great diffusing.

Question: Essences seem to be more *yin* in comparison with *qi*, is that right?

Elisabeth Rochat: Essences can produce liquids, but essences and *qi* produce all the movement of circulation and animation in the body, and all vitality can be understood by essences and spirits, or blood and *qi*. Nothing happens except through the dialectic effect of compenetration.

Claude Larre: Your question brings up a very important point. We are always eager to have all the material under our scrutiny, which is not how it is. Heaven exists, earth exists, your food is on the table and your wine is in the bottle, and what you want to do is see how it works. You need to find a way to speak about the process, forgetting heaven and earth, the food and the bottle because the process will apply to the materials concerned. This is the difference between the way the Chinese write and the way the westerner does. The Chinese are only concerned with the process, but we want to have everything under our supervision. The Chinese want to see *how* something works, not what is working.

Body hair and mai join their essences, and consequently there is a circulation of qi to the storage place (at the centre of the chest). The essences which are stored there manifest themselves as the shining radiance of the spirits. This shining radiance is stored in the four zang, and the qi returns to the judge.

Elisabeth Rochat: The meaning of this is that the lung masters the exterior zones of activity on the body, in other words the skin and body hair, and the essences and *qi* from the lung create this movement. The heart masters all the network of animation and all circulation goes through the network of animation. We know that the lung stores *qi* and the heart masters blood, and this forms a couple between heart and lung which summons vitality in the form of *qi* and blood.

By the *qi* of the lung which is clear, pure and fresh and so on, the spirits of the heart can receive all the power for their shining and radiance. If the spirits which are inside the heart are shining then it is called *shen ming*, and the other four *zang* can benefit from this radiance of the spirits. This is the meaning of the sentence:

This shining radiance is stored in the four zang.

The storage place referred to is the sea of *qi* in the middle of the chest, and one commentary says:

The ancestral qi, zong qi (宗 氣), *is accumulated by the lung, and the radiance of the spirits shines out from the heart. When the qi is increasing its prosperity and power the spirits can rule and prosper, and if the spirits rule then all the zang can act peacefully and normally, and all is in perfect equilibrium, ping* (平), *and rhythm.*

So one of the great agents in this process is the lung. For this reason the statement that '*qi* returns to the judge' means that the judge is a place or a function or a person who is able to appreciate, or to weigh and judge, and perfect equilibrium, *ping* (平), is achieved in this place where *qi* can be judged. This place is the radial pulse on the lung meridian.

The following sentence reads:

At this place the man who knows can determine if the patient is moving towards death or life.

This is one explanation of why one of the most important and special pulses, the radial pulse, occurs on the lung meridian. It is because the lung is in connection with the heart in order to ensure the perfect state by which the spirits can radiate and shine, and illuminate all the *zang*.

THE LUNG AND THE QI IN OTHER NEI JING TEXTS

Elisabeth Rochat: In a quotation from Su wen chapter 9 we can find another presentation of the relationship of the lung and the *qi*, and chapter 9 emphasizes the relationship between the lung and the heart.

Heaven nourishes man by the five qi. Earth nourishes man by the five tastes. The five qi enter by the nose and are stored in the heart and lung, and when they rise the five coloured aspects shine out correctly and the noises and notes resound.

The first question is what are these five *qi*? Are they the five odours or the five atmospheric or climatic agents? Odours, like tastes, come from the decomposition of things and beings, so why can the heart or lung not be nourished by odours? You know that odours are very important in all dietetic preparation! But some commentators very rightly say that odours come from the earth, from form and shape, and from things and beings of the earth, and these five odours are not properly from heaven. This text says heaven nourishes human beings by the five *qi*, and this means the five qualities of *qi* of heaven: wind, warmth, cold, humidity and dryness. These five qualities of *qi* actually reach a person, structure, constitute, and restore them, and each has a particular affinity with one of the five *zang*. But odours and atmospheric agents come with respiration by the nose, which is the orifice of the lung. These particular five qualities of *qi* of heaven come with respiration, enter and penetrate through the heart and lung and then go to the five *zang* and into the whole circulation of *qi* in a person. Afterwards, as a result, the five coloured aspects shine out because the heart is strong and firmly established. The five colours show especially on the face which has a special connection with the heart, and the heart masters the network of animation and especially the network carrying blood. If good quality blood is carried by a network of animation full of force then your face will have good colour.

Notes and noises resound because the lung is strong and also firmly established. The lung masters the *qi* and is also the organ which ensures the power of all sounds that come from a person. So this is another example of the relationship between heart and lung at the level of respiration and the penetration of the *qi* by which heaven nourishes.

Su wen chapter 11 says :

The stomach is the sea of liquids and grains.

The stomach is called the sea of liquids and grains because from this sea essences and *qi* can overflow into the other *zang*, as we saw in Su wen chapter 21. The stomach is sometimes the great fountain for the six *fu*.

The five tastes enter by the mouth and are stored in the stomach in order to nourish and maintain the qi of the five zang. The mouth of qi is on the tai yin.

The mouth of *qi*, *qi kou* (氣 口), is the name of the radial pulse. The mouth is like an opening or an orifice, or an harbour where something converges in order to enter or go out. It is like the mouth of a river, and at this place on the radial pulse the *qi* just appears.

The explanation of this quotation is that the stomach alone cannot diffuse and propagate the essences which come from digestion, it needs the transportation of the spleen, and the spleen is in very close relationship with the lung. We saw this in the processing of liquid foods, and in the meridian *tai yin* which unites spleen and lung with the same quality of *qi*. It is also from the lung that essences and *qi* can be diffused and propagated throughout the body. For this reason the quality of *qi* coming from alimentation can be seen through *tai yin*, especially through the lung because the lung not only receives the essences coming from alimentation but also, as we saw in Su wen chapter 9, the essences coming from heaven via respiration. At the level of the lung there is a junction between the essences and *qi* of heaven and earth, and the lung is also connected with the sea of *qi*, *tan zhong* (膻 中), ancestral *qi* and so on.

In addition, because of the relationship between the heart and the lung, on the *tai yin* meridian of the hand we have a very good place to judge the quality of *qi* and blood, and you can see the pathological alterations at every level, be it at the level of respiration, alimentation or the ability of making the spirits shine forth. All this is the reason why the radial pulse is so important. It is not the only possible pulse but it is definitely the most significant, and has been since the end of the Han Dynasty.

I would just like to mention the relationship of the lung to the nose. Ling shu chapter 17 says:

The qi of the lung is in free communication with the nose and through the nose. When the lung is in harmony the nose is able to perceive odours.

There is no difficulty here.

SU WEN CHAPTER 47:
THE SHAPE AND SIZE OF THE LUNG

Elisabeth Rochat: Ling shu chapter 47 discusses what your lung is like inside, and what the consequences of the tendencies towards certain syndromes are:

When the lung is small there is little liquid, there is no wheezing and panting.

This does not mean that the lung is too small, but just that the *qi* can be circulated easily and the liquids will not stagnate, if the *qi* is circulating with ease then respiration is good and there is no panting and no noise coming from any obstruction.

When the lung is big there is a lot of liquid and illness such as blockages in the thorax, closing at the throat, and qi moving in countercurrent can easily occur.

When the lung is big it means that it is too big and it tends to do too much and get blocked as a result. It also means that the opening and circulation are not good, and if the opening at the throat is not good it cannot ensure free communication, so all kinds of blockage and closings occur at the throat, for example sore throats.

When the lung is high and the qi goes up this causes panting and coughing.

When the lung is too high, as for example can happen when there is grief and the lung rises up, the movement upwards is too strong, and the *qi* goes up too high. This is called *shang qi* (上 氣). The *qi* is in a high part of the body but moving in countercurrent. As a result respiration is not good and there is panting and coughing.

When the lung is low it stays at the cardiac orifice and causes pressure on the liver, and you can easily have pains on the side.

This is because the cardiac orifice is the upper orifice of the stomach, and the communication between the stomach and the lung is not easy if the lung is too low. As a result there is a transverse countercurrent and the expanding, spreading out activity of the liver is disturbed, and the person can easily have pain in the area of the ribs.

When the lung is firm and strong there are no illnesses such as coughing or qi which rises up too much.

If the lung is firm and strong then the *qi* is strong and can easily be kept in its natural current.

When the lung is fragile there are bitter illnesses called xiao dan (消 癉).

Where internal heat leads to deterioration of the *jin* (津),

the fluids, and to wasting, the patient becomes very thin and is easily subject to attacks. When the lung is fragile it is easily dominated by the fire of the heart and you get this bitter illness. Bitter illnesses are ones which cause a lot of pain, and the text uses 'bitter' in order to make a subtle connection with the heart. Also, all these diseases come from fire and warmth. It is the action of fire on the metal, and it means that the interstitial liquids are easily destroyed.

When the lung is in a good state then there is harmony and ease and one is very rarely subject to attacks. When the lung is inclined to one side, then there are one-sided pains in the thorax.

In another part of Ling shu chapter 47 we find the same description for each of the five *zang*. For example, if the heart is too small or too large and so on, and afterwards there is a description of the exterior structure of the body, for example through the skin and the bones. Bones are obviously inside the body but they are also a sensible and perceptible structure, and they are exterior relative to the *zang*.

Su wen chapter 47 says:

If the coloured aspect is white and the texture or the structure of the flesh is small, then the lung is small.

The texture or structure of the flesh refers to all the structure at the superficial level of the body.

If it is very coarse and rough or loosely woven then the lung is very big. If the shoulders are strong and the lateral pectorals are very developed then the lung is high.

If the lung is high it is a sign that all the movement of *qi* is rising up too much and consequently the shoulders and upper part of the body are too strong.

If the axillary crease descends right down to the ribs then the lung is low. If the shoulders are in a good state and the back is well developed then the lung is firm and solid. If the back and shoulders are thin and feeble, then the lung is fragile. If the back (especially the high part of the back and the lateral parts of the thorax) is well developed then the lung is in a good state. If the ribs lean to one side and are separated (i.e. are very far apart) then the lung is inclined to one side.

PATHWAYS THROUGH THE LUNG

Elisabeth Rochat: Let us now look at all the pathways that pass through the lung. The network of animation of the *tai yin* of the hand, the lung meridian, rises from the diaphragm and takes its special relationship of belonging and dependence with the lung. The pathway then comes out at the level of the axillary crease.

The meridian of the large intestine comes into *que pen* (缺盆), Stomach 12, which is like a turn-table for many networks of animation. Afterwards it goes and takes its specific relationship of *luo* (絡) with the lung, and then goes down to the diaphragm.

The kidney meridian passes through the liver and diaphragm and then goes out in the middle of the lung and follows the pharynx. A branch of this meridian from the lung goes out and takes a *luo* (絡) relationship with the heart. It is quite interesting that there is a relationship between lung and heart through the kidney meridian!

The liver meridian comes out of the liver and passes through the liver and diaphragm and rises and flows powerfully into the lung.

The heart meridian from the connections of the heart, *xin xi*

(心 系), returns and rises to the lung. Afterwards it descends to the level of under the armpit.

As for the pathways of animation other than the meridians, amongst the *luo* we just have the great *luo* of the stomach, which we saw previously. Amongst the meridian divergences, *jing bie* (經 別), that of *tai yang* of the hand (small intestine) enters the lung and then goes to the heart. That of the *yang ming* of the hand (large intestine) goes from the large intestine to the lung in a relationship of belonging. Afterwards it goes up following the pharynx. The meridian divergence of the lung enters at the level of *yuan ye* (淵 液), Gallbladder 22, and goes into the depths of the body to the lung where it diffuses.

THE LUNG IN OTHER CLASSICAL TEXTS

Elisabeth Rochat: In certain pre-nineteenth century but post-Nei jing texts there are some interesting quotations on the lung.

The lung makes the qi come out and the kidneys make it come in. The lung is the one who has mastery over the qi, and the kidneys are the root of the qi.

So speaking of *qi* we are not to forget the kidneys and the original *qi*, *yuan qi* (元 氣), which are really the root of *qi* for all animation. For this reason in a symptom such as asthma it is very important to make the distinction between pulmonary asthma and nephritic asthma. If you have difficulty in expiration it is connected with the lung and if you have difficulty in inspiration it is connected with the kidneys. But obviously there are other symptoms and indications.

There is a quote from Hua Tuo, a great doctor of acupuncture from the second or third century AD:

The lung is the source of the qi of life, thus it is the flowery canopy for the five zang.

Flowery canopy, *hua gai* (華 蓋), is also the name of *Ren* 20, which is just at the level of the heart.

It covers all the zang.

Here the ideogram for covers is the same as that which specifies the action of heaven, it is a brooding movement like a hen which broods over her eggs.

It is empty like a hive and it has no orifice of communication or penetration towards the bottom. On inspiration it is full, and on expiration it empties. It directs transport and transformation of the clear and unclear. It is the bellows of the forge of the body of man.

LUNG PATHOLOGY IN THE NEI JING

Elisabeth Rochat: We can now see the main pathological tendencies of the lung and then look at the descriptions of the lung syndromes in the Nei jing.

The lung masters *qi* and guides and leads inspiration and expiration, thus its pathology will mainly show a disturbance and countercurrent in the movement of *qi* through respiration. Su wen chapter 74 says that all kinds of precipitation and agitation in the breath which cause obstruction and blockage are dependent on the lung. The main symptoms are coughs with countercurrent movements of the *qi*, panting, swelling and blockage in the area of the thorax and ribs. Or it could be that there is not enough *qi* to ensure good respiration, and its force is not enough.

We can also make a distinction between fullness and emptiness. In fullness with internal causes the lung is unable to propagate and make *qi* circulate correctly. The *qi* is blocked in the heights, and the lung is animated by the movement of rising up. As a consequence the movement of pressure to make things descend is not enough, and you get all sorts of symptoms dependent on that, with the *qi* moving in a countercurrent upwards.

With emptiness, the *qi* of the lung itself is insufficient. The traditional comparison is that ancestral *qi* is beating but like a drum without any force or real resonance. There are a lot of symptoms associated with this state of emptiness, for example all circulations are blocked because the *qi* of the lung is not enough. In Ling shu chapter 8 it says the nose can be blocked and cannot function, and all the *qi* and animation of *qi* in the body is diminished. About fullness of the lung, Ling shu chapter 8 says you have panting and thirst.

Another point is that the lung, mastering all the body's *qi*, receives the one hundred *mai* for the morning audience. Thus, when the lung is ill the repercussions are felt all over the body, and if the *qi* of the lung is diminished or weakening, or if the lung is too warm and the 'leaves' of the lung are burnt, then consequently the lung cannot make the *qi* circulate to give a gentle heat and humidification, and as a result there is a kind of impotence and flaccidity and a paralysis, the *wei* syndrome (痿). In this state the person becomes weaker and weaker, and the skin and body hair become burnt, lose their lustre and become brittle. In this situation you can also have a disturbance of the person's sweat. Sweat can flow out spontaneously because of the lack of balance between *yin* and *yang*, *qi* and liquids.

You can also have a great sweat during sleep which stops when you wake. This is the result of the emptiness of *yin*, because when the defensive *yang qi* goes into the depths of the interior during the night, if the *yin* is not sufficient to be compenetrated by *yang* they cannot join together, so the *yang* is forced out and you get this kind of sweat. When you wake and the defensive *qi* returns to the level of the skin and is sufficient to close the pores, the sweat stops. All these signs of disturbed sweat are indications that the rhythm at the exterior level of the skin is not operating well, so consequently all kinds of perverse *qi* can attack easily.

We saw that the main function of the lung is *qing su* (清 肅), the movement of oppression which makes things descend. The lung is like heaven in this because it has very clear *qi* which is able to ensure this pressure. If this function of the lung is disturbed, the circulation and regulation of the waterways is upset, and transport to the bladder and the bottom of the trunk is not good. You can have stagnation and blockage of liquids, a quantity of phlegm and pathological liquids. If this is serious, in some diseases of the lung you can also have a kind of oedema. If any of the other viscera is ill this can have repercussions on the lung because the lung receives all the *qi* of the organism. The best example of this is the cough, because although coughing is linked with the lung, each of the viscera can be the cause of a cough. So to treat the cough we have to carefully consider not only the lung but which specific syndrome is involved.

PATHOLOGY IN LING SHU CHAPTER 30

When perverse qi, xie qi (邪 氣), *is in the lung you get the following illnesses: layers of skin are painful, the person has chills of cold and fevers of warmth alternating, qi rises in a countercurrent and the person pants, sweats and coughs with their shoulders and back moving.*

Elisabeth Rochat: The explanation is not very difficult because the same movement is found in the lung and the skin, and if the perverse *qi* attacks this movement which is in the lung then the movement of the skin cannot be good, and of course all the *qi* and essences which go from the lung to the skin are not good. So for this reason the layers of the skin, the superficial part of the body, are painful. Also if the lung is attacked by the perverse, the circulation is not good and harmony between *yin* and *yang*, particularly at the level of the defensive and nutritive *qi*, is not good.

If defence and nutrition are not in a good state sometimes they can resist the perverse and sometimes they can not. Sometimes cold is stronger and sometimes warmth is stronger, and you get alternating chills and fevers. Then because the lung itself is disturbed the *qi* rises up in a countercurrent and you have panting and sweating because the *qi* is not able to ensure solidity at the level of the skin. You get a cough with the shoulders and back moving because there is a blockage in the breathing. Some commentaries say that if the perverse *qi* is in the meridians you can have this kind of cold and warmth together, and you will often have a headache at the same time. But if the perverse *qi* is only in the *zang* and not in the meridians you will have warmth and cold without headaches.

The treatment for all this is that you have to puncture the points at the level of Lung 1 and Lung 2. The text here does not give the names of the points but only the locations. They also give the location of the *yu* point of the lung, Bladder 13. Some commentaries, especially modern ones, interpret the text to mean the *yu* of the heart and the *yu* of the lung. Another point which is indicated is Stomach 12, *que pen* (缺 盆), to expel the perverse. But some commentaries say that if you puncture this point too deeply you can cause a countercurrent in respiration.

PATHOLOGY IN SU WEN CHAPTER 2

When the lung is ill there is panting, coughs, the qi is in countercurrent, there is pain in the shoulders and in the back, There is sweating, pain in the coccyx area, pain in the medial aspect of the thigh, pain in the knee, pain in the back of the femur and the calves.

Elisabeth Rochat: All these are symptoms of fullness, and panting, coughing, *qi* in countercurrent, pain in the shoulders and the back and sweating are a result of the obstruction or blockage of the *qi* of the lung with the countercurrent rising up. As a result all the networks of animation, especially carrying blood, are blocked in the upper regions of the trunk. The movement of oppression and descending is not enough, and the stomach which is also responsible for the descending movement does not have the participation of the lung, and the liquids of the stomach are not able to descend normally. The liquids are expelled by the *qi* which is blocked, and they go out in the form of sweat because the rhythm of opening and closing at the level of the skin is not well regulated. The particular areas of pain mentioned on the calves, coccyx and so on are, I think, the points of junction with other meridians such as the kidneys and bladder.

The connections between the *tai yang* of the foot (bladder meridian) and the lung are very clear. The *tai yang* of the foot masters the *biao* of the body, and like the lung has a special relationship with the external area of the body, so it is implicated during an attack of perverse energy.

PATHOLOGY IN SU WEN CHAPTER 22

In the case of emptiness qi is diminishing so it can no longer ensure respiration and the person has a buzzing in the ear and a dry throat.

Elisabeth Rochat: If the *qi* is diminishing it cannot ensure going out and coming in either, and for this reason respiration is not good. If the *qi* of the lung is not able to give a subtle stimulation and excitation through the circulation, perverse *qi* can come in and you get this kind of buzzing in the ear because there is not enough *qi*. The throat is dry because if the *qi* is not sufficient liquids cannot be produced or circulated. The treatment is on the *tai yin* of the hand. Some commentaries suggest Lung 8. The bladder and kidney meridians are also used according to some commentaries. For example Kidney 7, *fu liu* (復 溜), and bladder points to expel the perverse *qi*. Some other commentators, especially modern ones, indicate treatment on the *jue yin* (厥 陰) of the foot, the liver meridian, because the lung meridian is the first in the whole circulation and the liver meridian is the last. If you treat them both together then you can have an effect on the total circulation of *yin* and *yang* of the twelve meridians.

APPENDIX

THE LUNG FROM THE NEIJING JINGYI

The lung is located in the middle of the thorax, *xiong zhong* (胸 中). Its main meridian runs along the larynx and goes out, it descends and has a *luo* (絡) connection with the large intestine, it also has a *biaoli* (external/internal) relationship with the large intestine. The parts of the body with which it is linked, *he* (合), are the skin and body hair, its orifice or opening is at the nose.

Its functions are to master the *qi*, *zhu qi* (主 氣); to direct expiration and inspiration, so as to ensure the reciprocal communication of the *qi* from the inside and outside of the body, to receive the one hundred *mai* in morning audience, thus distributing the power of its fullness, *chong* (充), to the whole body; to master, *zhu* (主), the skin and body hair as well as the moistening and irrigation of the flesh. Its *qi* is in free communication, *tong* (通), with the nose which can thereby smell odours.

1. The lung masters the *qi*, *fei zhu qi* (肺 主 氣).

The *qi* represents what is essential for maintaining the vital animation of the human body. Its origin is twofold: on the one hand from the essential *qi*, *jing qi* (精 氣), that derives from the liquids and grains that form solid and liquid food, and on the other hand from the *qi* of nature that enters the body through inspiration.

That 'the lung masters the *qi*' means that the *qi* of the human body is under the mastery of the lung. The *qi* of nature which is outside the body enters it through the inspiration of the lung. The *qi* coming from the digestion of grains which are inside the body passes, *jing* (經), by the *mai* (脈) of the spleen to be transmitted and transported, *chuan shu* (傳 輸), and rise and pour out into the lung. The two kinds of *qi* unite and join together, accumulating in the middle of the thorax, *xiong zhong* (胸 中), at the sea of *qi*. This is called *zong qi* (宗 氣), ancestral *qi*.

The ancestral *qi*, *zong qi* (宗 氣), goes out of the larynx to produce inspiration and expiration, it connects with the *mai* of the heart to diffuse and spread, *bu san* (布 散), throughout the whole body.

For this reason the meaning of the expression 'the lung masters the *qi*' is not only that the lung masters expiration and inspiration but also that it masters the *qi* of the human body that rises and descends, that is in *biaoli* exchange (i.e. that goes towards the interior or towards the exterior). All of this is also under the mastery of the lung. Thus it is said in Su wen chapter 10:

All the qi is dependent on the lung

2. The lung has the charge of minister and assistant, *xiang fu* (相 傅). It governs well-regulated rhythms, *zhu zhi jie* (主 治 節).

Minister and chancellor, *xiang fu* (相 傅), indicates the one who assists the prince and master, *jun zhu* (君 主).

Well-regulated rhythms, *zhi jie* (治 節), designates the physiological activities that ensure the constant maintenance of the functions of the *zang fu.*

In the human body every kind of organism and function can therefore rely on well-regulated and ordered activities. Although the heart has the role of governing the *shen ming* (神 明), the radiance of the spirits, nevertheless it receives support and help from the lung. When heart and lung are well-regulated, then the whole vital ensemble takes place normally, correctly and without disorder.

So, in Su wen chapter 8 it says:

The lung has the charge of minister and chancellor, from it stem well-regulated rhythms.

The lung's function of being minister and chancellor appears most clearly in the relationship between the *qi* and the blood. The heart masters the blood, the lung masters the *qi.*

It is thanks to the circulation of *qi* and blood, which ensures the movement for transporting food, that the human body can maintain the mechanism of each organism, thus ensuring their own vital functions and their mutual relations are fulfilled as normal.

The transport and circulation of blood, although under the authority of the *qi* of the heart, nevertheless needs the *qi* of the lung to be able to spread out everywhere with ease, and it is by connecting with the *mai* of the heart that they communicate freely everywhere in the whole body.

Thus Ling shu chapter 71 says:

It is thus that the ancestral qi, zong qi (宗 氣), *accumulates in the middle of the thorax, goes out of the larynx, to connect with the mai* (脈) *of the heart and gives rise to expiration and inspiration.*

Heart and lung, blood and *qi*, help each other, and it is their close reciprocal relationship that ensures their functioning.

3. The *qi* of the lung descends, *fei qi su jiang* (肺 氣 肅 降). It ensures the communication and regulation of the waterways, *tong tiao shui dao* (通 調 水 道).

The circulation, transport and evacuation of fluids, *shui ye* (水 液), which concern each organism in the human body are not only related to the spleen's function of transporting, *yun* (運), but are also closely related to the lung's function of governing descending, *su jiang* (肅 降). The *qi* of the lung descends, *su jiang*, (肅 降) and the water pathways by which the waters move, *shui dao* (水 道), can communicate freely and descend to the bladder. Thus it says in Su wen chapter 21:

The liquid and solid food enter the stomach. They float and overflow into the essential qi. Above they are transported to the spleen, the qi of the spleen diffuses the essences, which rise to reach the lung and ensure the communication of the water pathways. Below they are transported to the bladder.

If this descending of the *qi* of the lung loses its normality there can be a rising in countercurrent which causes gasping, *chuan* (喘), and coughing, *ke* (咳). When this has repercussions on the water metabolism it can result in a stopping or stagnation of these liquids, and when it is intense, the urine no longer flows and there is formation of watery swellings, *shui zhong* (水 腫), a kind of oedema.

For this reason, the correct or incorrect functioning of the urine is closely related to the lung's function of descending the *qi*. It is because of this that in later times the lung was called the upper source of liquids.

4. The lung masters the skin and body hair, *fei zhu pi mao* (肺 主 皮 毛).

The lung masters spreading. On the exterior it is linked to the functions of the skin and body hair. This appears especially in the following two aspects:

The lung masters the *qi*, directs respiration, ensures that there are mutual exchanges between the *qi* of the interior and the exterior of the body. The pores (literally the holes of the sweat) of the skin also have the role of diffusing the *qi*. This is why Su wen chapter 3 calls the pores the doors of the *qi*, *qi men* (氣 門).

On the other hand, the skin and body hair rely on the warming and moistening which are provided for them by the lung so that they are well irrigated. If the *qi* of the lung diminishes and weakens it can no longer distribute the *qi* to warm the skin and body hair. Then the nutrition of the skin and body hair is insufficient and there is emaciation and wasting, drying out and withering.

Thus it says in Ling shu chapter 10:

When the qi of the tai yin of the hand is interrupted, the skin and body hair are burnt.

LUNG PATHOLOGY

PRINCIPAL CAUSES OF DISEASE

1. The six perverse influences, *liu yin* (六 淫)
Cold, made worse by wind
Dryness, made worse by heat

2. Internal attacks
Damage to the lung *qi* through:
Longstanding and chronic illnesses
Excessive tiredness leading to exhaustion of lung *qi*
Dietary disturbance, where there is repercussion on the lung from an attack on the spleen and stomach
All kinds of disorders linked with water, dampness, phlegm and the unclear

3. The seven emotions, *qi qing* (七 情)
Sadness, *bei* (悲), blocks communication and destroys the *qi*
Oppression, *you* (憂), slowly weakens the vitality

PRINCIPAL SYMPTOMS

Cough, *ke sou* (咳 嗽), (from external injury or internal attack)

Dyspnoea, asthma, *xiao chuan* (哮 喘), (from emptiness or fullness)

Phlegm, *tan* (痰), (which can be cold or hot, and combined with damp, dryness or wind)

Pain in the thorax, *xiong teng* (胸 疼), (from blockage of *qi*, stagnation of blood, phlegm and dampness, or emptiness in the *mai*)

Spitting of blood, *ke xue* (咳 血), haemoptysis (from emptiness or fullness)

Loss of voice, *shi yin* (失 音), hoarseness, (from emptiness or fullness)

PRINCIPAL PATTERNS

1. Patterns of perverse fullness of the lung:
Wind and cold constrain the lung, *feng han shu fei* (風 寒 束 肺)
Perverse heat attacks the lung, *xie re fan fei* (邪 熱 犯 肺), which can be subdivided into the following different headings:

> Wind and heat attack the lung, *feng re fan fei* (風 熱 犯 肺)
> Fire and heat, *huo re* (火 熱), in the lung
> Phlegm and heat obstruct the lung, *tan re yong fei* (痰

熱 壅 肺)

Phlegm and the unclear block the lung, *tan zhuo zu fei* (痰 濁 阻 肺)

The perverse influence of dryness injures the lung, *zao xie shang fei* (燥 邪 傷 肺)

2. Patterns of perverse emptiness of the lung:

Emptiness of lung *qi*, *fei qi xu* (肺 氣 虛)

Emptiness of lung *yin*, *fei yin xu* (肺 陰 虛)

The lung loses its regulation and free circulation (of the water ways), *fei shi tiao tong* (肺 失 調 通)

INDEX

INDEX